WELLNESS AFTER STROKE

A holistic fitness guide with daily workouts to keep you moving!

Dr. Sarah Stollberg, PT, DPT

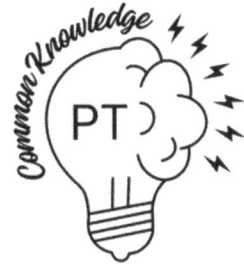

New Orleans, LA, USA

The information provided in this book is intended for general informational purposes only and is not a substitute for professional medical advice, diagnosis, or treatment. Always seek the advice of your physician or other qualified health provider with any questions you may have regarding a medical condition.

Before starting any exercise program or making significant changes to your diet, it is crucial to consult with your healthcare provider to ensure that the chosen activities and dietary modifications are safe and suitable for your individual health needs and conditions. This is especially important if you have pre-existing health concerns, injuries, or if you are pregnant.

The author and publisher of this book are not responsible for any specific health or allergy needs that may require medical supervision and are not liable for any damages or negative consequences from the use of the information provided herein. The exercises and nutritional guidance should be approached with caution and individual responsibility.

Participating in physical activities and following dietary recommendations involve inherent risks of injury or adverse effects, and individuals engage in such activities at their own risk. The author and publisher disclaim any responsibility for any injuries or health issues that may result from individuals following the information in this book.

It is essential to listen to your body, progress at a safe pace, and make modifications to the exercises or dietary recommendations based on your personal abilities and limitations. If you experience any discomfort, pain, or other symptoms during or after following the guidance in this book, it is advised to stop the activity immediately and consult with a healthcare professional.

By reading and using the information in this book, you acknowledge and agree to the terms of this medical disclaimer.

© 2024 Common Knowledge PT, LLC

Designed and Published by Common Knowledge PT, LLC. All rights reserved.
Illustrations by Sarah Stollberg.
Icon graphics licensed through Canva.com.

No part of this publication may be reproduced, distributed, or transmitted in any form or by any means, including photocopying, recording, or other electronic or mechanical methods, without the prior written permission of the publisher, except in the case of brief quotations embodied in critical reviews and certain other noncommercial uses permitted by copyright law. For permission requests, contact the publisher.

Paperback ISBN: 979-8-9900976-2-9
Spiral Bound ISBN: 979-8-9900976-0-5
E-PUB ISBN: 979-8-9900976-1-2

Common Knowledge PT, LLC

New Orleans, Louisiana
United States of America
www.CommonKnowledgePT.com
commonknowledgePT@gmail.com

TABLE OF CONTENTS

I. Introduction
Max Rehab Potential   **01**
The Role of this Guide   **03**
Joint Protection   **05**

II. Holistic Wellness
Physical Exercise   **10**
Nutrition   **12**
Sleep   **18**
Mental Health   **20**
Social Health   **23**
Wellness Checklist   **26**

III. The Exercises
Let's Get Moving!   **28**
Lying Down   **34**
Seated   **48**
Standing   **62**
A Note About Balance   **75**
Energy Shot   **76**
Rest Days, Illness and Listening to Your Body   **77**
Make It All Matter!   **78**
Caregiver Notes   **79**

MAX REHAB POTENTIAL
People discharged from therapy may not feel ready.

Rehabilitation can be a long process, especially after a stroke. Many times individuals are discharged from physical or occupational therapy because they hit the *maximum rehab potential* but they may still be in the process of reaching their personal goals.

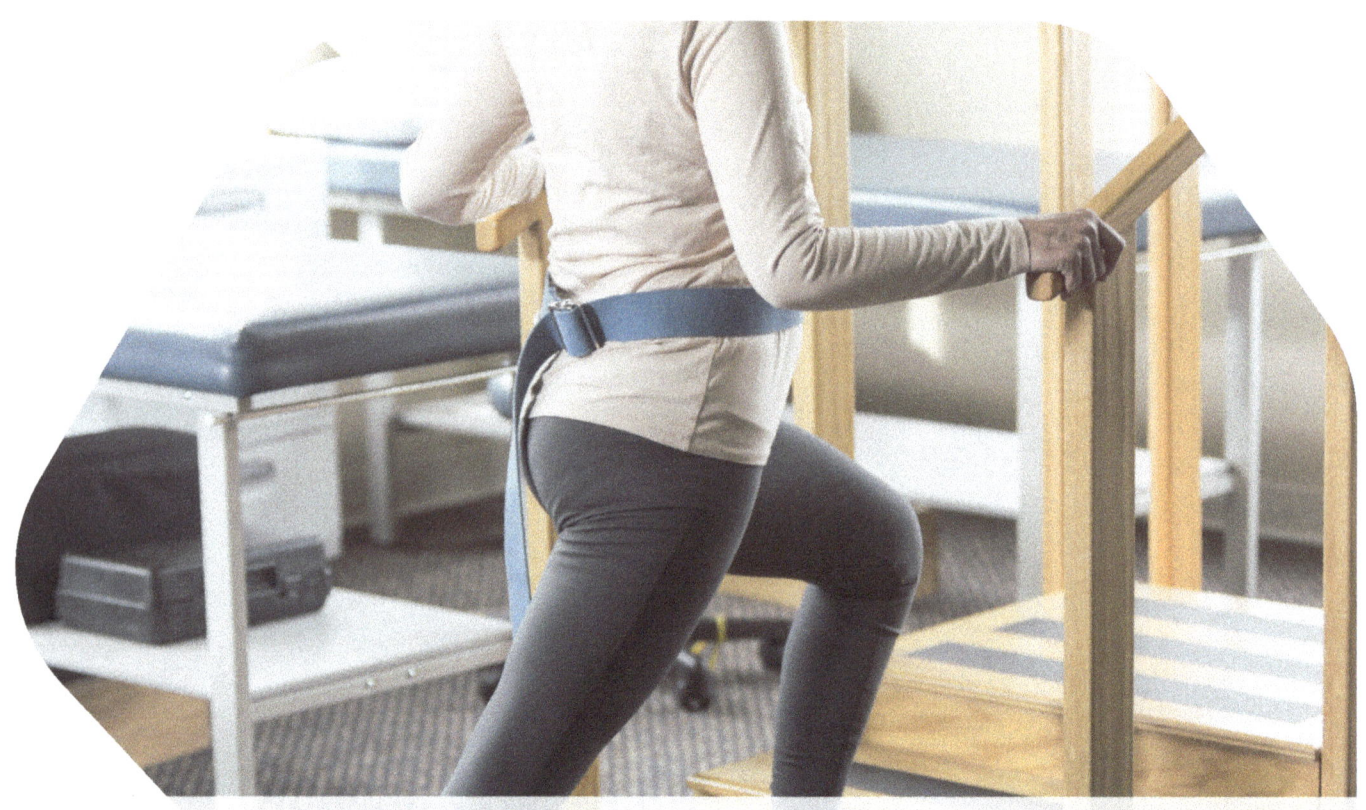

Just because formal therapy is finished, it doesn't mean your healing journey is over!

Why did they discharge me if I'm not back to 100%?

There are many reasons you may be discharged from therapy. In the United States, insurance limitations can be a factor. Insurance companies can set a specific number of approved visits regardless of the individual case. Some insurances focus on specific measures that may not accurately reflect your progress or status. The definition of what is "medically necessary" as opposed to wellness services, which are not a covered therapy benefit, can be a grey area. Copays and deductibles may also limit your ability to attend ongoing therapy. Regardless of the insurance company, they typically don't approve endless therapy sessions.

Insurance is not the only limiting factor. Regardless of insurance, the nature of therapy in a clinical setting is acute or subacute. It is designed to address a specific injury or deficit, then send you on to your daily life. The goal of therapy is always to transition to an independent wellness routine.

You may have other barriers to your therapy participation such as the time commitment required, having reliable transportation to and from therapy, or other ongoing health issues.

Finally, we must acknowledge that the limiting factor, at times, is the lack of motivation. Therapists use physical exercises to drive you toward your goals; but just as important is the education they provide. Education includes what to be doing throughout the 165+ hours a week you are NOT in therapy sessions. You must be motivated to do the home exercises and make adaptations which the therapists recommend, or there will not be progress. When a person is not retaining information or is not motivated to follow through with the activities prescribed, discharge is often earlier. The person is, knowingly or not, self-limiting any further potential **at the moment.** There are many factors that contribute to this but talking with your therapist about any barriers is the best way to overcome them.

Good thing for you is that you are motivated because you are reading this guide.

THE ROLE OF THIS GUIDE

Regardless of your goal status after therapy discharge, ongoing fitness and wellness is necessary to maintain or continue to progress in your function. This guide is intended to be used as your primary exercise routine, with tips and information regarding other aspects of wellness. It may have been prescribed to you by a therapist to get you started with an at home wellness routine, and needs to continue as a habit long after therapy has stopped.

The exercises are designed with the most common stroke presentation of one weaker side in mind. As with any generalized fitness plan, you need to listen to your body and modify or skip things as appropriate.

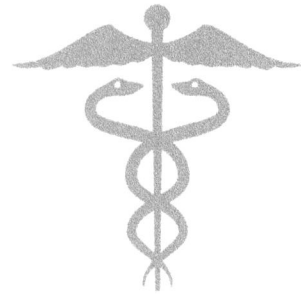

Before starting any new fitness routine, it is important to consult with a medical professional to ensure that you are healthy enough to participate.

By participating in this fitness routine, you acknowledge and accept that you are doing so at your own risk. You are responsible for your own health and safety during the routine, and the creator and publisher of the routine is not liable for any injuries or damages that may occur as a result of your participation.

WHO THIS GUIDE IS FOR

This guide is for those that have suffered a stroke and have completed or are near their physical or occupational therapy discharge but still feel like they have more potential.
This may also be for people who have had a stroke many years ago, have no new complications and are cleared by a medical professional to exercise. It is ideal for those intimidated by conventional gym settings or fitness guides that don't take into account long term, often one sided weaknesses.

WHAT THIS GUIDE IS NOT

This is not a replacement for traditional physical and occupational therapy. Each stroke is so individualized and there is no replacement for skilled, hands-on therapy. No matter how mild or severe the stroke, an evaluation with a therapy team is always recommended for initial care.

JOINT PROTECTION

It is my goal that you stay healthy and injury free during your workouts. That is why I want to point out the importance of joint protection! Following are the highest risk areas for joint instability, and thus injury after a stroke.

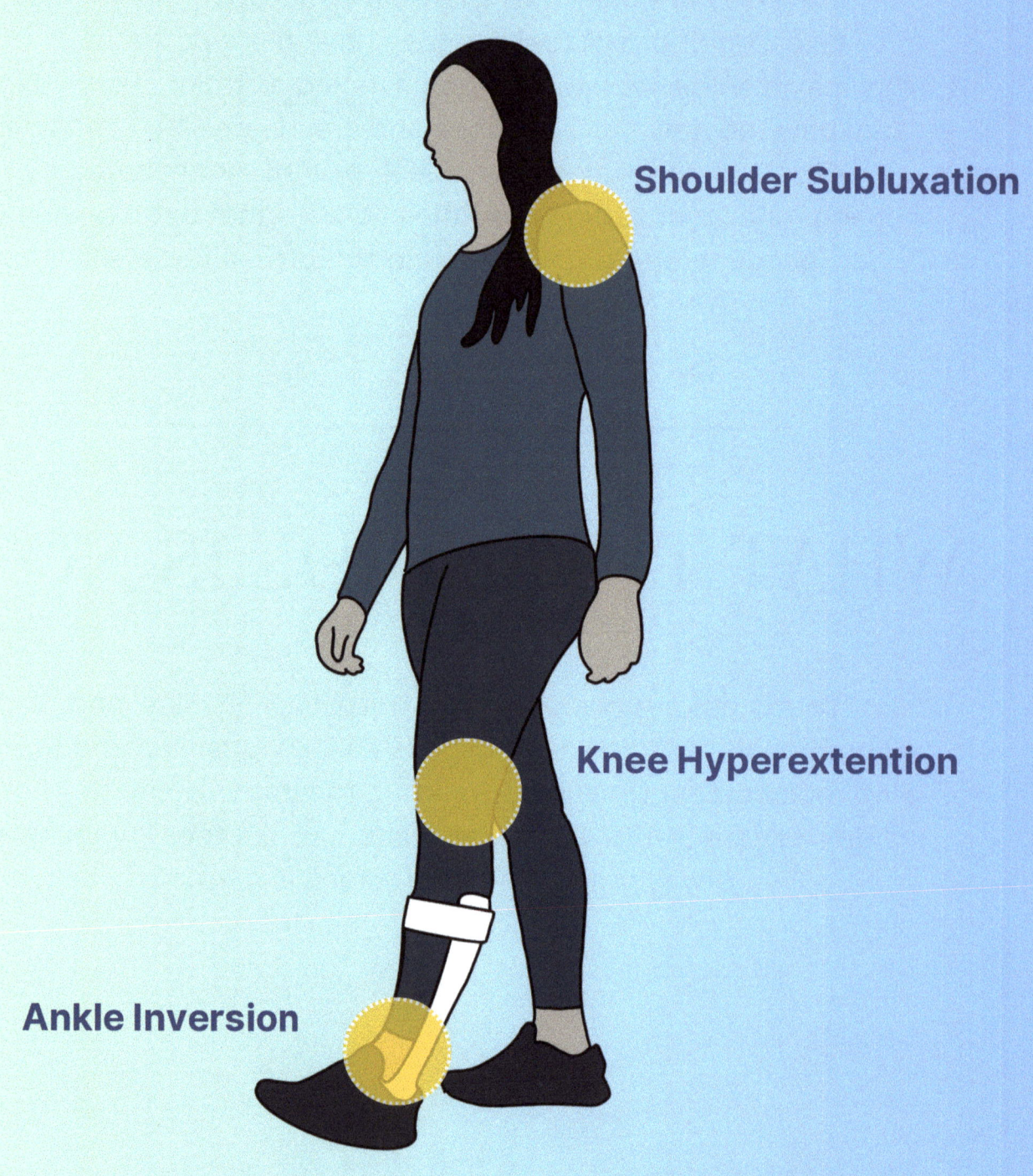

JOINT PROTECTION

Shoulder Subluxation

Often the supportive muscles of the shoulder, known as the rotator cuff, are significantly affected after stroke. This can lead to the muscles no longer holding the arm as tight into the shoulder joint socket. This results in a high risk for injury to the nerves and blood vessels that run through the arm, which can be painful.

Correct support and positioning of the arm is important to protect the shoulder from further injury. Unfortunately, traditional arm slings are not effective. Some slings are made specifically for subluxation and you can check with your medical providers to see if they are right for you.

When seated, make sure your affected arm is supported at the elbow by an armrest, table top, pillows, or your lap. Do not let your affected arm hang down to your side. Never let anyone pull on your affected arm, which risks creating or worsening a subluxation.

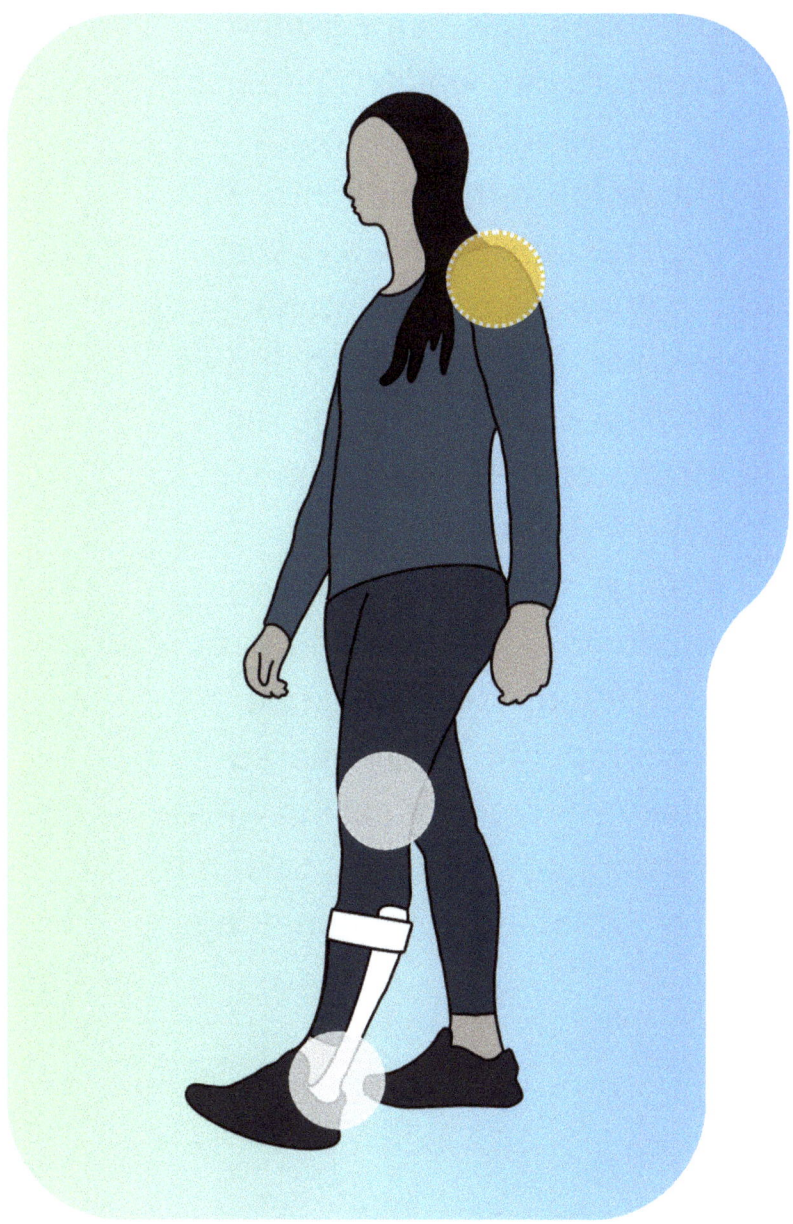

JOINT PROTECTION

Knee Hyperextention

When the muscles that cross the back of your knee (the hamstrings) are weak, they are not able to support the joint and you end up relying solely on the ligaments of the knee for support. Under that much pressure the ligaments often stretch and allow the joint to "hyperextend", that is, bend back in a way the knee is not supposed to go.

Over time, this "wrong way" pressure can lead to knee pain or orthopedic problems. Never force the knee into hyperextension. Always stop the knee once straightened, not beyond, for straight leg moves. Be especially mindful during stretches to not press into hyperextension. This can be difficult to feel or control so watch your leg, using a mirror as needed. There are knee brace options on the market to minimize hyperextension while walking, but the best solution is strengthening your hamstrings.

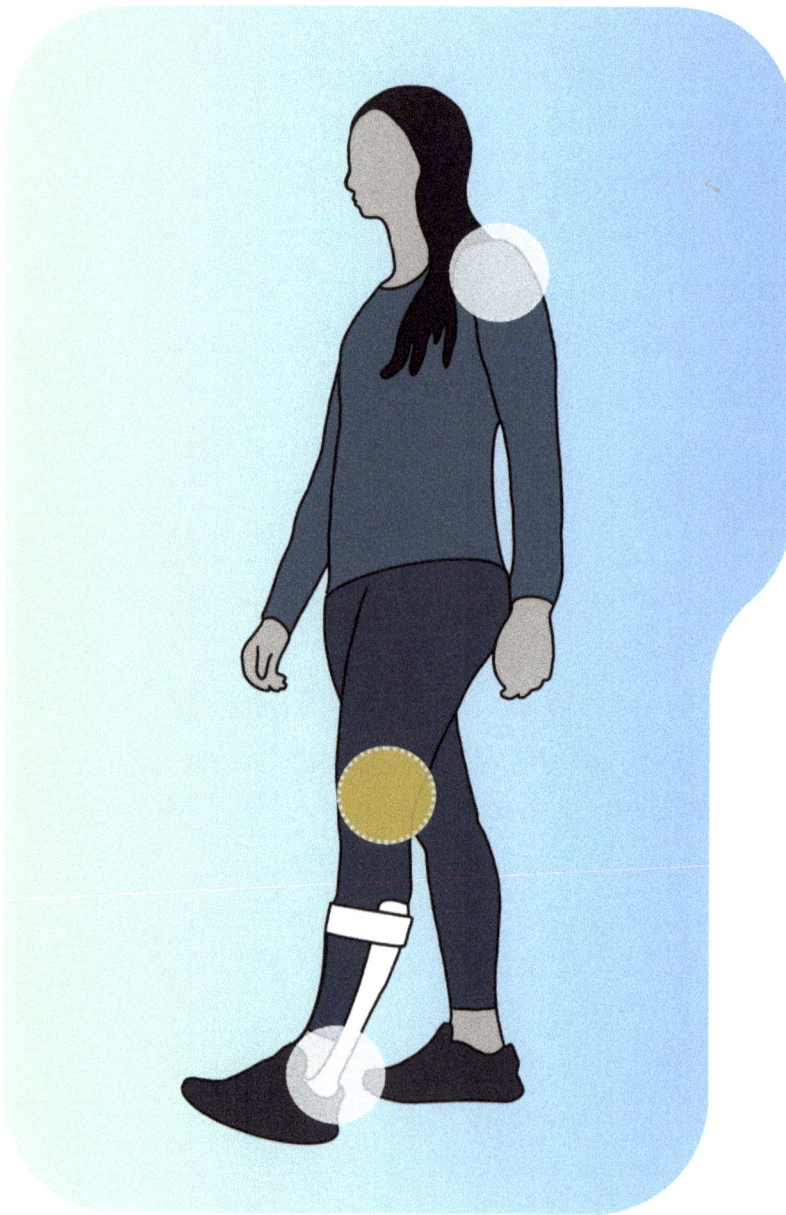

JOINT PROTECTION

Ankle Inversion

Ankle stability is critical to overall balance. Unfortunately, the ankle muscles are often the most severely affected leg muscles after a stroke. There are multiple muscles and factors involved, but with common presentations after stroke, the foot tends to point down and in. This leads the ankle to roll out, the motion most people think of for spraining their ankle. That is exactly what can happen when standing or walking after a stroke.

The best way to prevent this further injury is strengthening, but when that is gradual or not possible, proper footwear and bracing is important. Some people find a high top tennis shoe to be enough support. Avoid backless shoes and sandals. It can be helpful to wear an ankle foot orthosis (referred to as an AFO) or figure-8 ankle brace to keep your ankle more supported. Work with your medical professionals to determine which brace, if any, is appropriate for you.

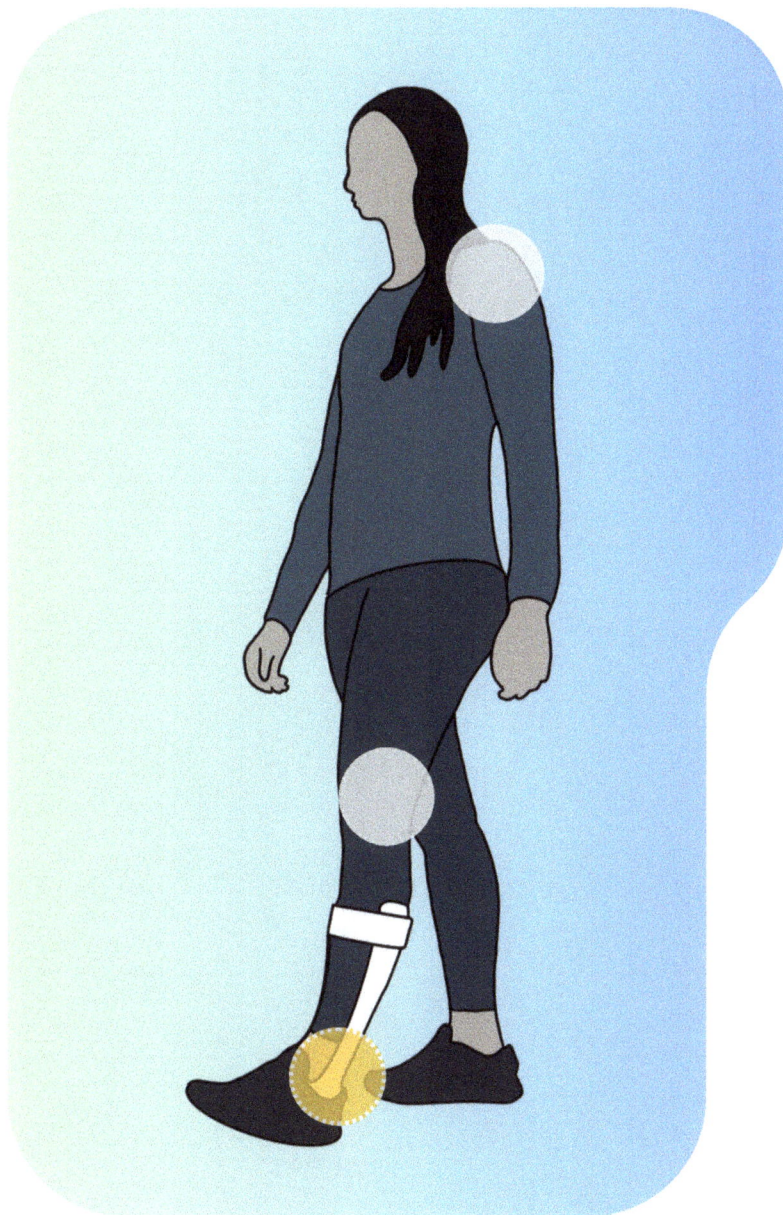

WELLNESS IS MORE THAN JUST PHYSICAL EXERCISE.

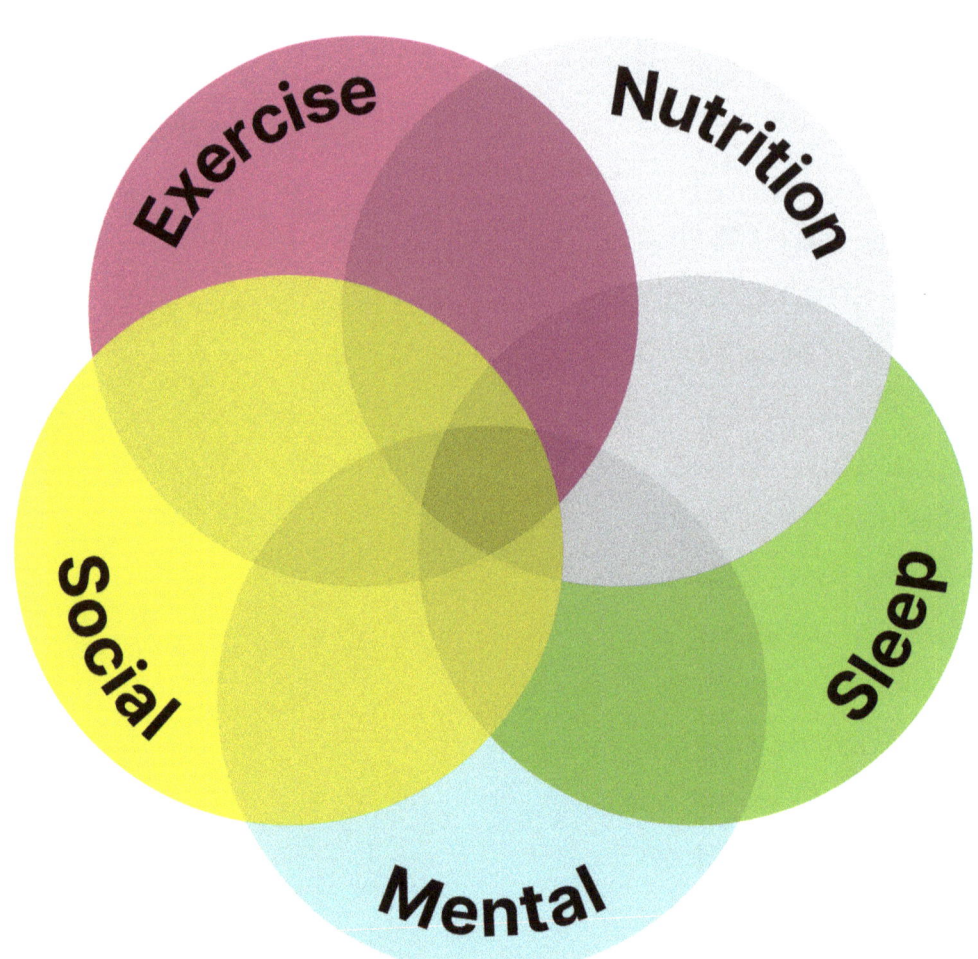

IT'S HOLISTIC.

PHYSICAL EXERCISE

Movement is medicine to the body. Our muscles, joints and brains need movement to thrive. Exercise helps increase oxygenation to the brain and helps with focus, sleep, memory, energy, and so much more. That is why physical exercise is the primary focus of this guide.

Cardiovascular Activity

In addition to the strengthening and stretching in this guide, aim to do some form of cardio 3-5 days a week. This could be anything that consistently keeps your heart rate elevated for 15-30 minutes. Great options are stationary bikes or brisk walking, if safe. Even self propelling in your wheelchair can be cardio. Do what you can!

If you have not been active, gradually work your way up to that goal time by starting at 5 minutes and adding 2-3 minutes as tolerated.

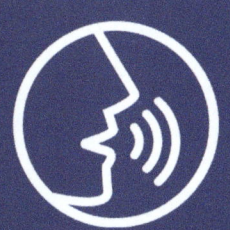

A good gauge that you are working at the right intensity is that you are breathing heavily but able to control it. If your speech is not affected use the talk test - you should be able to complete phrases but not full conversations without pausing to breathe.

Health Benefits of Walking

Standing and walking have so many health benefits beyond muscle and heart strength. Getting into an upright position improves breathing by creating more space for the lungs to expand, improves digestion and bowel function, can promote circulation to decrease swelling, and even helps control blood sugar. If you cannot safely stand or walk, you can still get some of these benefits by focusing on unsupported sitting with good posture and self propelling your wheelchair.

...but there is more to it than just movement!

HOW WELL DO YOU KNOW YOUR BODY?

After having a stroke, frequently checking your blood pressure is a MUST!
Use an at-home electric cuff for easy monitoring. Let your doctor know if the numbers are out of recommended ranges and do not start an exercise session if your systolic (top number) is over 180 or diastolic (bottom number) is over 100.

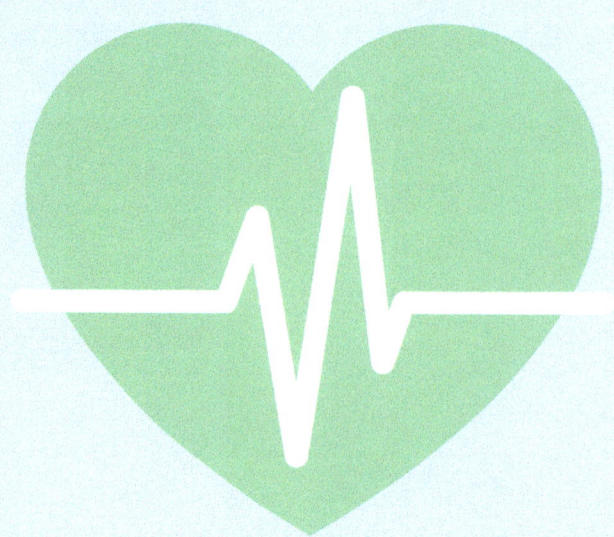

Current technology makes it much easier to keep track of our vitals and movement. Take advantage of the features on your smart phone or smart watch for tracking heart rate, steps and more. Ask if digital monitoring is offered by your medical team.

NUTRITION

This is not a diet or meal plan book. I am not going to tell you exactly what to eat or to count calories. It is however important to understand the basics of how to fuel your body.

You are what you eat is true! To build muscle and sustain muscle you need to ensure you are getting enough lean protein in your diet. Current recommended amounts of protein according to the Mayo Clinic are 0.8g/kg body weight for the average sedentary adult. After the age of 40-50, that increases to 1-1.2g/kg. Keep in mind general recommendations are based on maintaining your current physical status. If you are trying to build muscle (which most of us are), eat at least 1g/kg of your goal body weight regardless of age.

I did the math for you:	Adult under 50 years old 0.8g/kg body weight	Over 50 years old 1-1.2g/kg body weight
120 lbs	44g	54-65g
170 lbs	61.7g	77-93g
230 lbs	83g	104-125g
280 lbs	102g	127-152g
330 lbs	120g	150-180g

For reference, a 4 oz chicken breast is 35g of protein
a cup of 2% milk is 8g of protein
a large egg is 6g of protein

Protein is a priority, but not the only nutritional factor.

Real Foods

There is a lot of research surrounding the health implications of the processed food that is so prevalent in American and worldwide diets. Ultimately, eating REAL food is better for our bodies than eating heavily processed food. Most packaged foods, even those claiming to be "healthy", have been so processed and repurposed that they no longer hold the same nutritional benefits as their whole counterparts. To simplify this, think about a home cooked meal of baked chicken breast and chopped and roasted vegetables. Simple, yet each item starts in your kitchen as a single ingredient. The same processed freezer meal of chicken and vegetables has been broken down and re-combined with a variety of oils and chemicals to preserve it, retain textures, and create appealing colors. After eating it you are less full than eating the real version, have ingested notably more chemicals, sodium and sugars, and likely have less energy.

Easy guidelines to improve your healthy food choices are as follows:
- The less packaging the better.
- Choose ingredients you can pronounce.
- Vegetables in any form are better than none (fresh, frozen, canned).

Sugars and Fried Foods

We all know processed sugars and fried foods are not the healthiest choice. Try to limit these to only occasional and eliminate all sugary drinks from your daily routine. Pay attention to how you feel next time you eat a heavily processed meal or high sugar snack. The sluggish crash afterwards affects more than just your body in that moment, it affects your activity patterns day after day.

The combination of lean protein and a variety of vegetables, along with lowering your intake of sugars and fried foods will make a huge difference in your energy levels and your body's ability to build and sustain muscle.

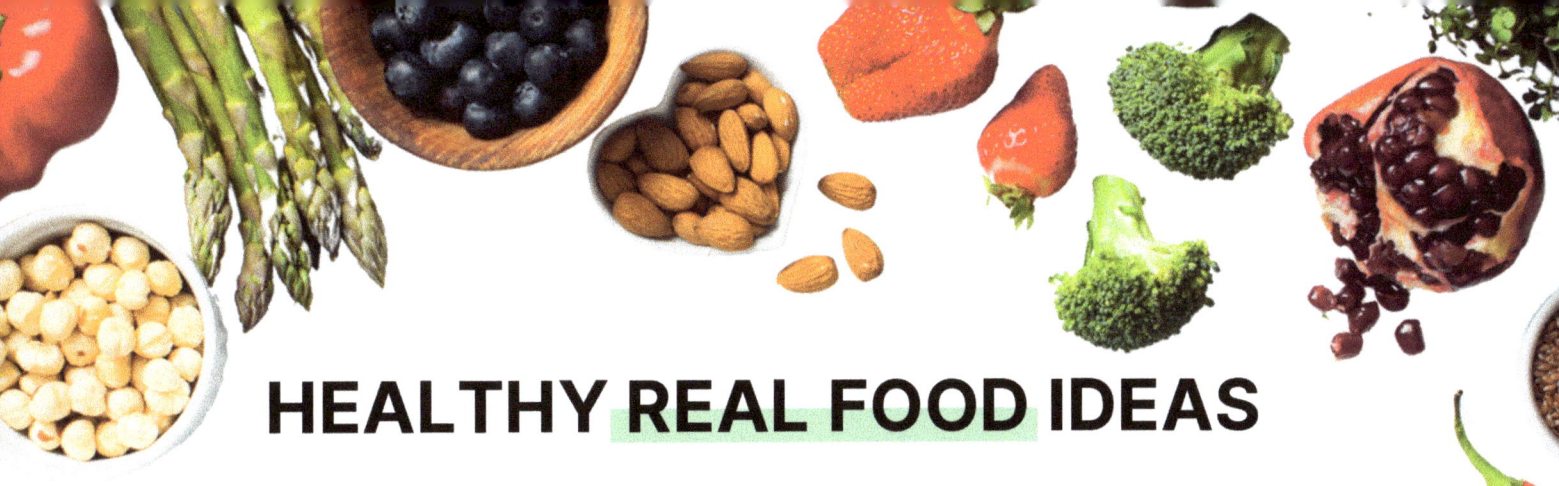

HEALTHY REAL FOOD IDEAS

Chicken Breast
Salmon
Ground Turkey
Lean Beef
Eggs
Chickpeas
Beans
Tofu

Whole Fruits
Leafy Greens
Whole Vegetables
Nuts
Cottage Cheese
Yogurt
Milk
Olive Oil

Be mindful of any swallowing difficulty post stroke. If you have any difficulties, follow recommendations from your speech therapist. Whole foods can be blended into smoothies if needed and protein powders can be added to supplement.

A NOTE ON WEIGHT LOSS

If you are currently overweight, weight loss can help make movement easier. However, initial focus on NOURISHING the body is most important. A starving or nutrient lacking body can not thrive. Focus on eating for strength and moving more; the weight loss will follow.

> **IF YOU CHANGE NOTHING ELSE, DRINK MORE WATER!**

WATER INTAKE

Water is the lubricant of our body - it keeps all things running smoothly. Imagine running a car for years low on oil - the gradual wear and tear destroys it. Same thing goes for dehydration. The body cannot function optimally without water.
Recommended water intake is about 15.5 cups (3.7 liters) of fluids a day for men; about 11.5 cups (2.7 liters) of fluids a day for women. The old adage of 8 glasses a day generally will be adequate for most adults.

And because it is such a common excuse... avoiding water so you don't have to go to the bathroom as much is not okay.
If that is how you feel, you need to assess what your barriers are for safe toileting and work with your family or caregivers to find solutions. It may be a urinal, in room commode, setting up a schedule to use the bathroom, or seeing a pelvic health physical therapist. Once you become consistent with hydration, your need to urinate will level out as your body adapts.

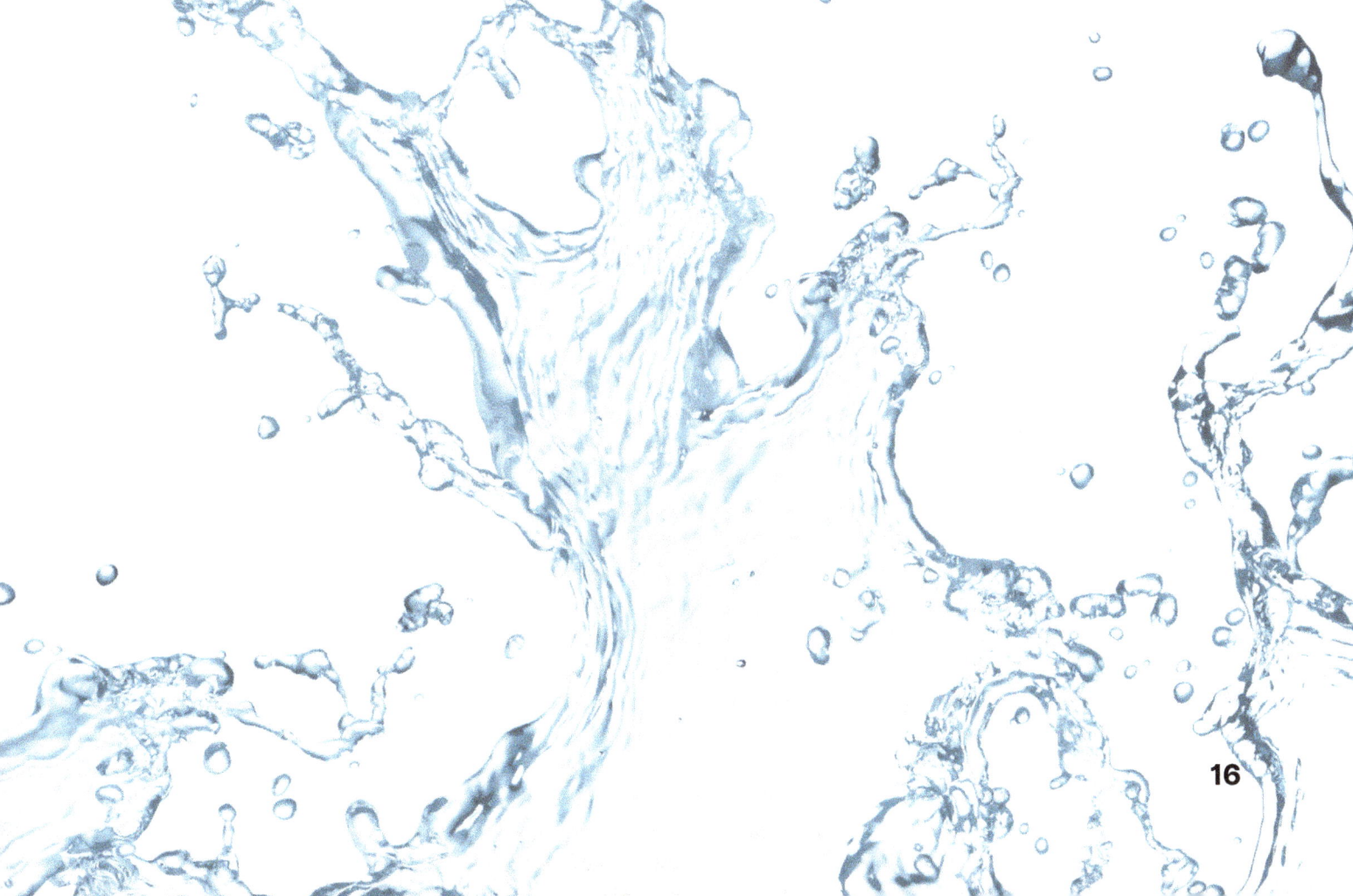

Alcohol

Alcohol is dehydrating to the body, affects our balance and motor control, and impairs cognition. None of these effects are beneficial to anyone, much less someone after a stroke. Alcohol can also increase your risk for stroke or recurrent stroke through side affects related to high blood pressure and diabetes. As with sugars and fried foods mentioned earlier, it is best to eliminate or limit alcohol from your regular intake. Seek further medical assistance if you feel your drinking is problematic and you need help stopping. There are many resources available online and within local communities to assist you.

Smoking

Everyone knows that smoking is not healthy. That doesn't mean everyone chooses to be mindful of that or is able to easily quit. If you are a smoker, it may have been a factor in the cause of your stroke. It is important to be aware of how continuing to smoke affects your body after a stroke so you can take the steps to quit.

According to the Stroke Foundation, being a regular smoker puts you in at least **twice the risk** of having a stroke, **three times the risk** if you are over 60 years old. Chemicals from smoking enter the blood stream and affect the consistency of the blood - making it thicker and sticker - thus at more risk to clot. The chemicals also promote build up of fatty plaques on the blood vessel walls making them narrow and hard - putting you at more risk for a blockage and also for a blood vessel to rupture. Good news is that research shows immediate benefits to stopping smoking after just one day, and benefits continue for over 20 years.

If it were easy to quit, it would not still be such an issue in our society's health. Just as with any other medical conditions, seek resources to help you achieve your goal to quit. There are many smoking cessation programs throughout the country and world. Many insurance companies or employee health benefits include smoking cessation programs.

SLEEP

Sleep is when our bodies are most active at regeneration and recovery. Making sure you have quality sleep is just as beneficial as good physical activity and healthy eating.

Most people do not realize that fatigue is a common symptom after a stroke. Your body has gone through a massive event internally and is using a lot of energy to heal.

Fatigue does generally improve over time after a stroke but by making sure your rest periods are truly that - restful - will help along the healing process.

Pain and Positioning

Often pain, spasms, or the inability to get positioned comfortably affects your sleep after stroke. If this is true for you, look over the following considerations:

- Time pain and spasticity medicines with your bedtime to improve falling and staying asleep. Make sure you stay within prescribed guidelines and talk to your prescribing doctor for specifics.

- Stretching your most spastic muscles before bed can help decrease intensity of spasms, decreasing the likelihood of it waking you later.

- Use pillows and wedges to get comfortable. Sleeping on your back or with your affected side up is typically the most comfortable annd be sure you have a pillow to support the arm and leg.

TIPS FOR BETTER SLEEP

Do not drink caffeine 10 hours before bedtime.

....

Keep daytime naps to less than 45 minutes.

....

Stop screen use (phones, TV) at least 1 hour before bed.

....

Avoid large, heavy meals 2 hours prior to bed.

....

Stay consistent with your wake and rise times 7 days a week.

Sleep tight!

MENTAL HEALTH

This guide is by no means a replacement for any form of mental health care. This is a reminder of how important it is to assess your mental health and reach out for help if needed. Having a stroke is a major life change and no one is expected to go through this alone. Depression and anxiety are extremely common after stroke. Please reach out to your healthcare provider for mental health resources if needed. Many insurances cover mental health services and there are many online and over the phone options you can access in the privacy of your home.

You can't fix a problem you don't know you have. Recognizing common factors that can negatively affect your mental health is the first step to improving your outlook.

Isolation

Usually, after a stroke your daily routine completely changes. You may no longer be going to work, running errands, or going to social events. That creates physical isolation. Deficits to your speech and ability to communicate can create cognitive isolation. It may also feel like you are alone in going through this event as your friends and family go on with their life as before. That isolation can make you spiral and decrease your motivation to move and participate with activities. Just know you are NOT alone. Working through these barriers can lead to a very fulfilling life going forward.

 **Be careful with social media!** It is easy to sit at home and compare ourselves to other people's "perfect lives" they post. No one is perfect. Consume only the media that is positive to you. Unfollow the rest.

Fear, Anxiety and PTSD

Having a stroke is a traumatic event both physically and emotionally. It is normal to be fearful of another stroke, movement that could harm you, or anxiety about uncertainties of your future. If the fear and anxiety are limiting you from daily activities, please seek professional help.

Stigma

The barrier of a stigma after stroke is real, both from yourself and the people around you. The assumption that you are now "disabled" can lead people to treat you differently as wrong as that may be. People less familiar with stroke may simply be unaware of what you ARE capable of. YOU may be unaware of what you are capable of. Break the barrier by showing people you are still you. Communicate to the best of your ability and educate those around you what you can do and what accommodations you may need. People are scared of what they do not know, so educate them. People are generally good; they want to help but do not always know how.

Cognitive Changes

Stroke is an injury to the brain - your command center - so yes, it can absolutely affect your cognition depending on the area of the brain affected. Figuring out what you still are good at and interested in gives you further purpose and mental stimulation. After a stroke, you may have difficulty finding words, difficulty understanding what other people are saying, and have memory challenges just to name a few. This can be extremely frustrating and can lead to a sense of helplessness. Figuring out your best form of communication and strategies to help memory with help from family, caregivers and your Speech Therapist can lead to the most independent outcome.

Lack of Support

Not having the physical, financial or social support you need can wear you down. Having community and help makes a world of difference to your outlook. See the Social Health section on page 23 for further explanation and take advantage of national and local resources. A local social worker with your healthcare system can be a great starting point.

All the barriers above are real feelings that should not be ignored but acknowledged. (It's OK and normal to feel these!) They shouldn't be your only feelings, though. There is no easy fix for any of these but the key is communication. Sharing your fears and concerns with those around you is the best first step towards a healthy outlook.

Stress is a huge barrier to healthy lifestyles

Here are some strategies to help immediately decrease stress responses and improve your outlook:

- Meditation

- Visualization (Visualization is a technique often used for relaxation or improving physical performance since an actual neural connection can be tracked to the area of the body you are visualizing. It can also be used to help motivate and set goals.)

- Pray or seek spiritual grounding

- Call a family member or friend

- Get outdoors - fresh air and nature is therapeutic!

- Listen to music

Our mind is our strongest tool - use it!

SOCIAL HEALTH

You are not defined by any one part of your medical history.
You are a daughter, son, sister, brother, mother, father, spouse, mentor, etc. You may be a business owner or an employee. You have hobbies and interests. These things combined with your values and personality make you, YOU. Not a medical diagnosis. These roles can feel like and likely have changed drastically since your stroke. But it is important that you find roles to continue to fill.

Finding a Role

It may start small such as folding laundry, or reading bedtime stories. It could be a new job or volunteering. This will be different for every individual. The main point is to find purpose. Finding purpose can directly and indirectly improve your health in other aspects. It can motivate you physically to move more, it improves your mental health, and can help strengthen and build social relationships. Below are some examples of in home and out of home roles to kickstart you but the list is endless.

Household roles
- Folding laundry
- Meal planner
- Unload dishwasher
- Feeding a pet
- Collecting the mail
- Light gardening

Family/social roles
- Being a friend and provide a listening ear
- Being the family comedian
- Parenting - no matter how old children are they need advice and guidance.

Work roles
- Resume your prior work if possible.
- Online or remote work in your area of expertise or hobby.
- Volunteer positions at local organizations.

If this is an area where you feel you are struggling, I challenge you to identify at least 2 roles that you are currently fulfilling in your life. Next, list 2 more roles to strive to fill within the near future.

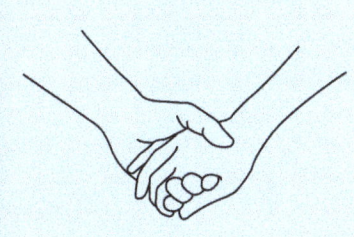 **If you have a partner, they may feel like more of a caregiver than a partner right now. Find small moments to get back to that feeling of partnership. It may be just holding hands, a compliment, or reminding them of a favorite memory.**

Having a sense of community can do wonders for your health.
Reach out to your core friend group if you feel that has distanced. A lot of people want to give "space" while you heal or they just do not know how to help. Be the first to reach out to get the ball rolling. Do not overthink it. Scheduling lunch or coffee with a friend is a great start. If swallowing is a deficit of yours and eating or drinking in public gives you anxiety, start with a non-food focused visit like walking (or wheeling) around a local park, or just a front porch meet up. You can also seek out local support groups, church communities, or fitness groups. You will be surprised how much your world will expand and outlook can improve.

If using a wheelchair or communication device means you could participate with that morning coffee group you used to attend, why are you not using them? Empower yourself by taking advantage of equipment and assistive technologies to rebuild social connections. I promise your friends want to see YOU, more than they care what you are sitting on.

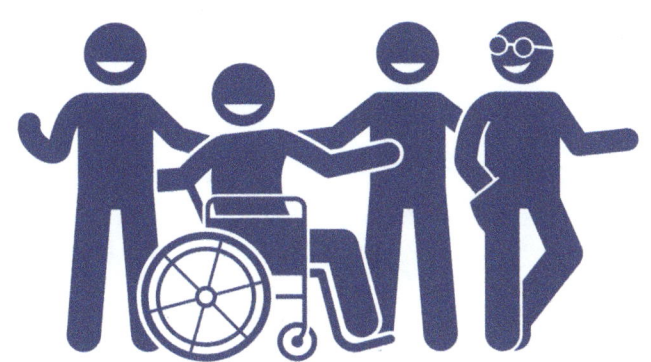

Communication limitations can largely impact your social interactions. This is one reason why it is so critical to work with a speech language pathologist for not only rehabilitation of speech but for alternative communication strategies.

Quality adaptive equipment is worth it!

If you are spending most of your time in a wheelchair please make sure you are in a good quality one! Proper support and positioning affects posture, musculature, pain (a.k.a. minimizing it), breathing, speech, swallowing, social interaction and mood!

Compare the following two scenarios:
1. You are slouched looking down, leaning to your affected side and your arm is dangling off (which is making your back and shoulder hurt). You are unable to self propel your manual chair and have to ask every time you want to move around the room.
2. You are sitting upright looking forward, centered in your chair with your affected arm supported and have a power joystick to be independent with where you move.

- In which scenario do you think you feel better?
- Which one are you more likely to want to talk to a friend?
- Which one would you interact with a waitress to order your own food?

Posture and position matter!

Finances and insurance affect what chair you are "given" out of the hospital but this is an area to be proactive and advocate for the best you can afford, even if it means more paperwork, or reaching out to charities, churches, or crowd funding to obtain it.

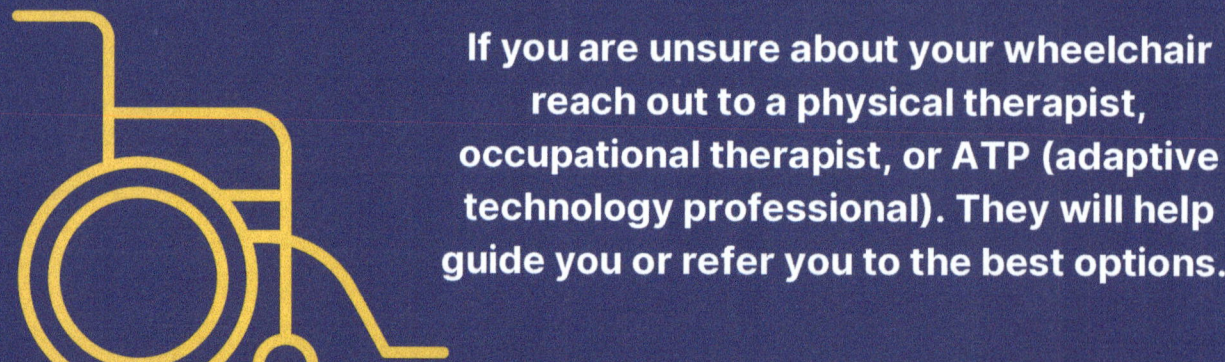

If you are unsure about your wheelchair reach out to a physical therapist, occupational therapist, or ATP (adaptive technology professional). They will help guide you or refer you to the best options.

WELLNESS CHECKLIST

PHYSICAL HEALTH   ☐ Follow the exercises in this guide 3-5 days a week.

☐ Focus on protein and vegetables. Eat fried foods and sweets sparingly.

☐ Prioritize water!

☐ Regular blood pressure checks.

☐ Good sleep habits.

MENTAL HEALTH   ☐ De-stress daily: meditate, visualize, pray, get outdoors or listen to music!

☐ Seek professional help if needed.

SOCIAL HEALTH   ☐ Identify 2 roles you currently fill.

☐ Set goals for 2 additional roles to fill.

☐ Find your community and reach out!

DON'T WORK TOWARDS THE PAST. WORK TO BE THE BEST VERSION OF YOURSELF NOW AND IN THE FUTURE.

THE EXERCISES

Let's get moving!

For ease of use, these exercises are broken down first by position they are done in. Regardless of your mobility level, there are exercises that you can complete. Work in your safe position! As you progress, you may work up to sitting or standing exercises. If you are already able to stand you can still benefit from the exercises in other positions. Listen to your body and be safe. Falls don't help anyone. Consistency with exercises that are moderately challenging is the goal, not wearing yourself out completely.

The schedule: If you have not been consistently exercising, start with completing the routine 3 days a week. The goal is to work up to 5 days a week consistently.

Every position focuses on a stretching portion and a strengthening portion. If you have time to stretch before and after each session I highly recommend it for best results and to keep soreness at bay.

A note about tone and spasticity.
A general rule is that anything spastic or tight needs to be stretched the most. Areas that are low tone or flaccid should be moved within the normal joint range but no further. Refer back to the Joint Protection section previously covered. Slow stretches with long holds are more effective than quick and short stretches that can actually have the opposite effect than desired.

The exercises are created with both your affected and non-affected side in mind. There are multiple modifications provided for each move so you can adjust to a challenging level for each side. **This means you will likely be following one modification for your right side and a different modification level for your left side. That's okay, it is expected!**

WHAT YOU NEED

Recommended Equipment:

exercise band or ankle weights
(alternatives: time! You can complete all the exercises without any added resistance- just increase the hold time to increase challenge)

stretching strap
(alternatives: dog leash, belt, rolled towel or bed sheet)

light hand weights 1-5 pounds
(alternative: use filled water bottles or cans)

safe space to workout
If lying down, a firmer surface works best, but a yoga mat on the bed can work.
If standing, make sure to have a sturdy support within reach.

*Pro Tip: Keep your band tied in a loop if tying/untying is difficult one handed. Sit to place it around your knees and ankles.

I recommend you complete all sets and reps with no added resistance your first time to help gauge your current strength and safety with each move. If it is easy and you have no pain, add resistance to a moderate effort level. Remember, good form and control during movements is more important than higher weight numbers.

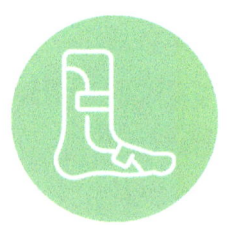

Note this bubble next to exercises that are appropriate to complete while wearing your AFO. You don't have to wear one with any of the exercises, if you have one, but certain exercises and stretches you cannot do wearing the AFO (due to need for further joint movement).

THE LEVELS

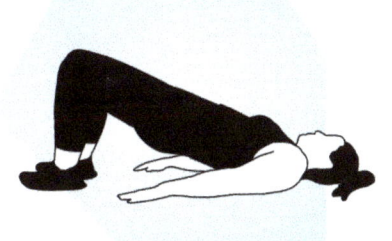
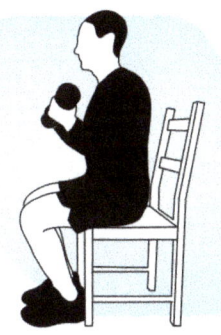

Lying Down
All exercises are completed either lying on your back, side or stomach (with modifications available). Only lay on the floor if you know you can get up! Try a bed or firm couch.

Seated
All exercises are completed sitting. You can complete these in a wheelchair (make sure it is locked!), or preferably a firm chair. Focus on sitting tall the entire time and try not to use the backrest.

Standing
All exercises are completed standing. Make sure you have something stable like a counter, railing, or heavy chair within reach if you lose your balance. Have a seat nearby to rest as needed.

If someone will be assisting you, have them read the caregiver tips on pages 79-80.

Warm up
For all levels it is great if you can do a short 3-5 minute warm up. This may be walking around the house or self propelling in your wheelchair with all available limbs to get the blood pumping.

Sets and Reps
All strength exercises are listed at 2 sets; this is a starting point. As you feel stronger and your endurance improves, you can increase up to 4 sets. It is also OK if your rep count varies anywhere between 8-12. Remember, focus on quality of the movement and use moderate challenge as your guide.

WHERE TO START?

As mentioned, performing these exercises in any position can be beneficial and you can definitely switch it up for variety - that's actually encouraged! But to help you decide where to start follow this simple flow chart.

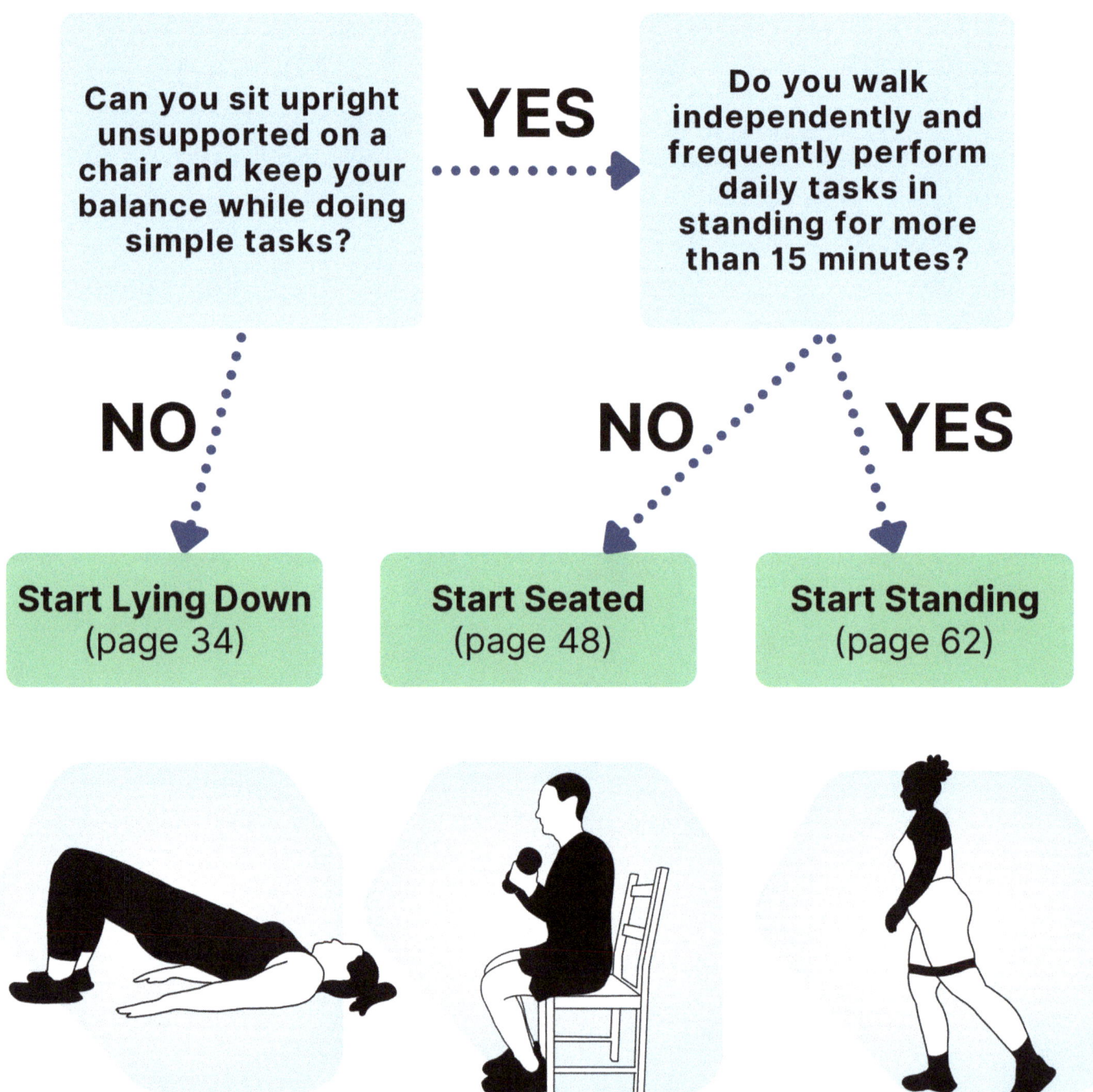

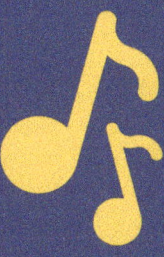

MUSIC - Turn it up!
Blast your favorite music to help motivate you and keep you focused on your workout.

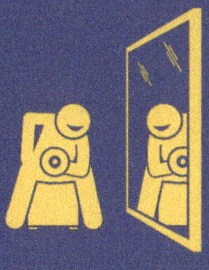

MIRROR
Exercising in front of a mirror can help give you feedback on the quality of your movements, especially since sensation is often affected after stroke, meaning it is harder to just "feel" how your body is moving.

MISSED DAYS
It's important to remember that consistency is key when building new habits. If you miss a day, don't beat yourself up about it. Just pick up where you left off and keep moving forward. Don't let guilt or false milestones hold you back from achieving your goals.

Leaving equipment visible increases the likelihood of working out!

Every exercise page includes tips and cues for proper technique in the circles.

- Read through the tips before you begin each move.
- It's like your very own therapist sitting next to you!
- If something is painful, check for adjustments or modify.

Modifications to make each move easier or harder are in the blue boxes at the bottom of each page.

Too Hard?
This option shows how to make the move easier while still working the same muscle group.

Too Easy?
You want a moderate challenge. This option shows how to make the move harder for the same muscle group.

LYING DOWN

LYING DOWN STRENGTH

Bridges

Hip Rotations

Straight Leg Raises

Biceps-Triceps Combo

Sidelying Leg Lifts

Sidelying Arm Lifts

Hamstring Curls

Shoulder Blade Squeezes

STRENGTH

LYING DOWN

Bridges

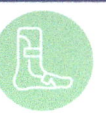

Start on your back with knees bent and feet flat.
Press into your heels and shoulders as you lift your hips.
Hold 3 seconds and then lower back down slowly.

Repeat 8-12 reps x 2 sets

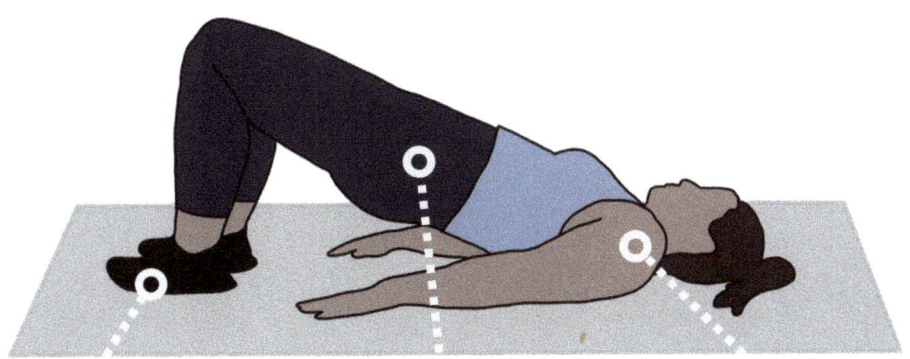

Feet sliding? Place a yoga mat underneath.

Stop when you make a straight line from knees to hips to shoulders.

Press into your shoulders, not your neck.

Too Hard?
Focus on core activation and tilting the pelvis but don't worry about lifting up yet.

Too Easy?
Increase hold time up to 10 seconds.

LYING DOWN

STRENGTH

Hip Rotations

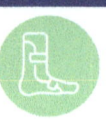

Start on your back with both legs straight, feet wide, and toes facing the ceiling. Performing one leg at a time, rotate your toes in toward the opposite foot. Pause then slowly return to the starting position.

Repeat 8-12 reps x 2 sets

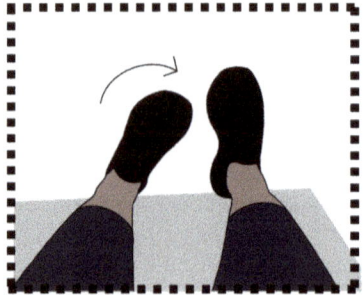

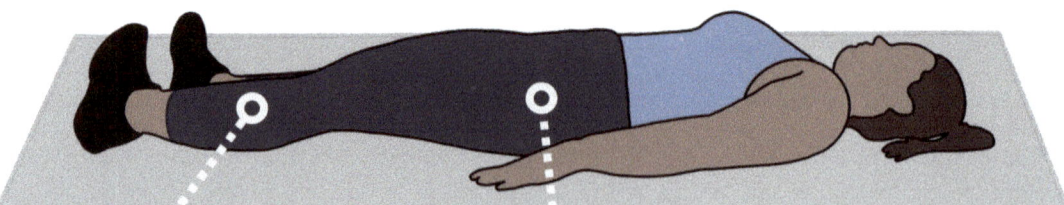

- Maximize benefit by trying to keep the ankle flexed and the knee straight.
- This movement originates at the hip. The whole leg should be rolling in.
- Try to rotate further each rep.

Too Hard?
Bend the opposite knee to help stabilize.

Too Easy?
Hover the leg off the mat, then rotate inwards. Lower after each set.

STRENGTH

LYING DOWN

Straight Leg Raises

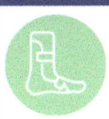

Start on your back with one leg straight and opposite leg bent.
Slowly lift the straightened leg 6-12 inches and pause.
Lower back down slowly.

Repeat 8-12 reps x 2 sets

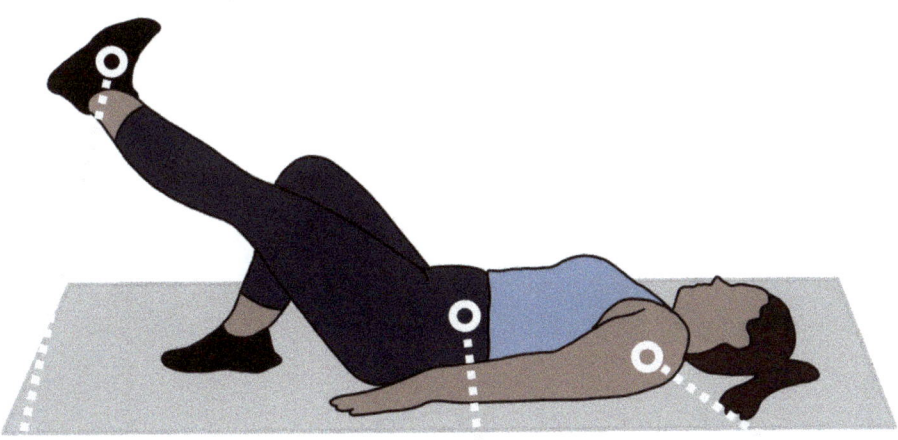

- If you can, keep the ankle flexed during the movement.
- Keep your core engaged and low back pressed flat - no arching.
- Focus on relaxing your upper body.

Too Hard?
Place a towel roll under your knee then straighten the leg.

Too Easy?
Add small circles before lowering your leg back down.

STRENGTH

LYING DOWN

Biceps-Triceps Combo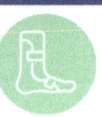

Start on your back with arms down at your sides. Bend one elbow to slowly bring your hand towards your shoulder. Slowly lower it back down and give extra effort at the end to straighten the elbow as far as it can go.

Repeat 8-12 reps x 2 sets

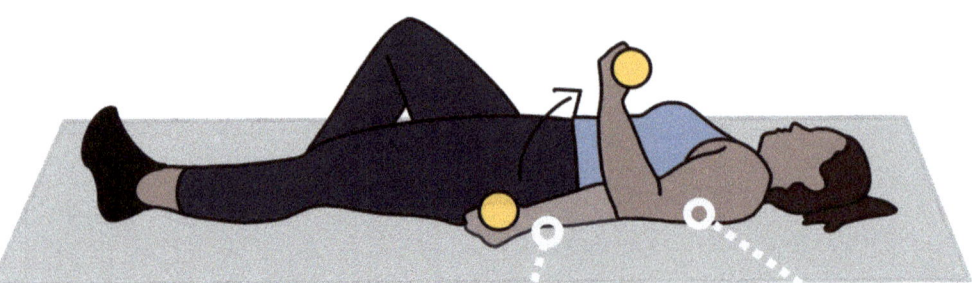

- Use hand weights as needed for adequate challenge.
- Don't let the hand sway side to side as you go - keep it centered.
- You want to feel a squeeze in the back of the upper arm as you straighten.

Too Hard?
Prop a rolled towel under the wrist to start the motion with an advantage.

Too Easy?
Add a punch towards the ceiling after bending your elbow.

STRENGTH

LYING DOWN

Sidelying Leg Lifts

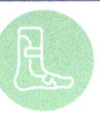

Start in sidelying. Keeping your top knee straight, slowly lift the leg towards the ceiling. Slowly lower to the starting position.

Repeat 8-12 reps x 2 sets

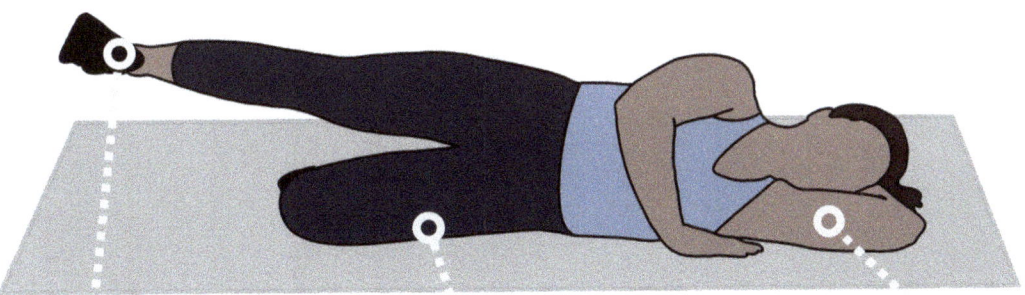

Keep the ankle flexed to maximize muscle facilitation.

Bend your lower knee to create a stable base.

Position your arms as needed for comfort.

Too Hard?
Perform the same move laying on your back - sliding the straight leg out to your side.

Too Easy?
Add front and back taps with your foot while lifting the leg.

STRENGTH

LYING DOWN

Sidelying Arm Lifts

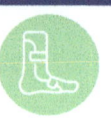

Start in sidelying with your arm as straight as you can along your side. Lift the whole arm up towards the ceiling 6-12 inches then slowly lower back down.

Repeat 8-12 reps x 2 sets

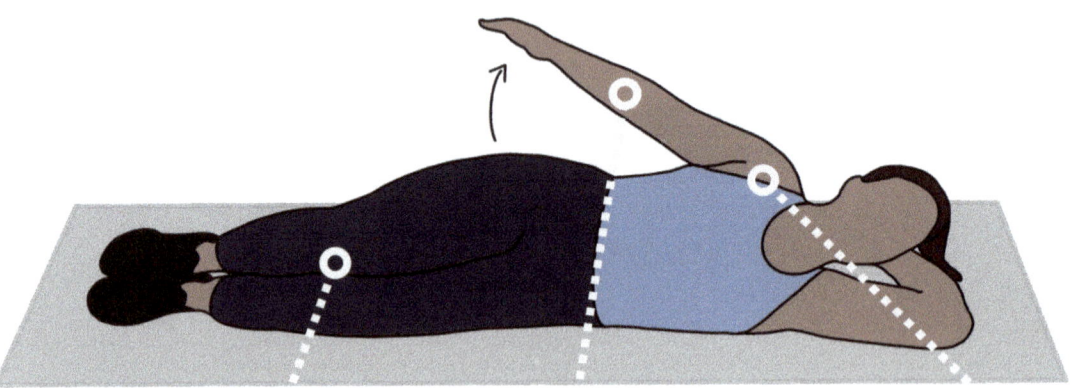

- Adjust your lower body as needed - bent knees will feel more stable.
- It's ok if you can't straighten all the way - do the best you can.
- Avoid letting your top shoulder sink forwards.

Too Hard?
Perform the move lying on your back. Slide your arm away from you to the side.

Too Easy?
Hold hand weights or hold at the top and add a palm up/palm down rotation with each rep.

STRENGTH

LYING DOWN

Hamstring Curls

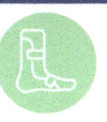

Start on your stomach. Bend one knee bringing your heel towards your buttocks. Slowly lower it back to the starting position.

Repeat 8-12 reps x 2 sets

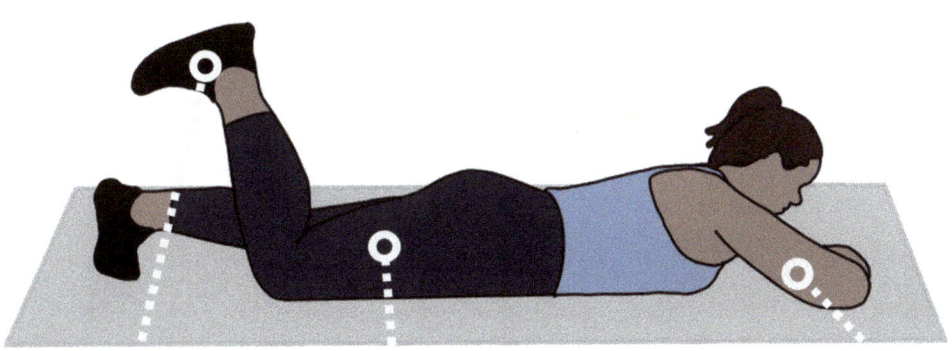

Keep the ankle flexed throughout the movement.

Don't let the leg sway side to side - keep it centered as it moves.

Position your arms however is most comfortable.

Too Hard?

Start with a towel roll under the ankle to begin the motion with an advantage.

Too Easy?

Add a band or weights at the ankles for resistance.

LYING DOWN — STRENGTH

Shoulder Blade Squeezes

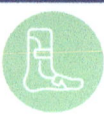

Start on your stomach. With both arms at your sides in a W position, slowly squeeze your shoulder blades together.
Hold up to 5 seconds then release.

Repeat 8-12 reps x 2 sets

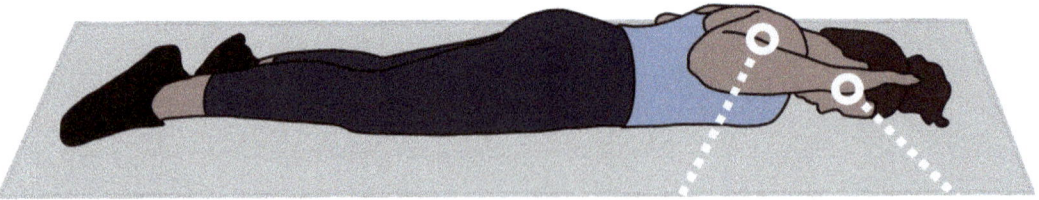

- If you cannot get to the W position, try both arms straight at your sides.
- Keep the shoulders depressed away from your ears the entire time.
- Use a towel roll at your forehead or lay your head to one side.

Too Hard? Perform the move lying on your back.

Too Easy? Extend arms to a V position or use hand weights.

Lying Down
Quick View

Bridges
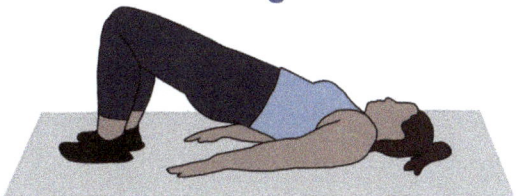

Hip Rotations
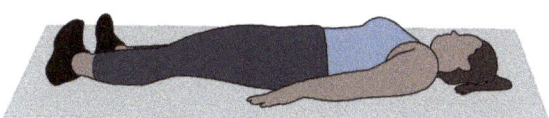

Straight Leg Raise
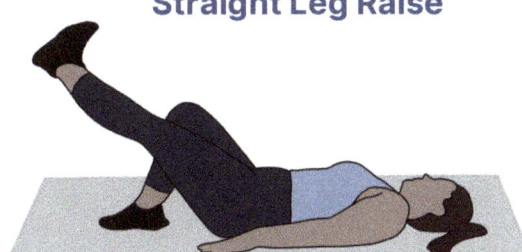

Biceps - Triceps Combo
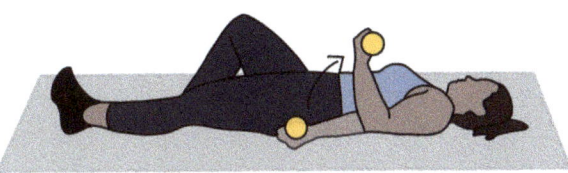

Sidelying Leg Lifts
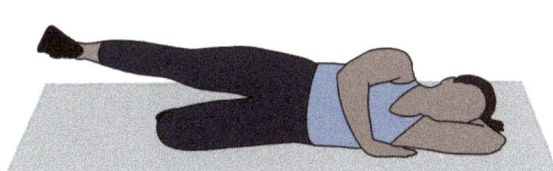

Sidelying Arm Lifts
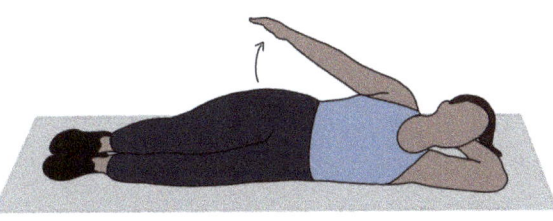

Hamstring Curls
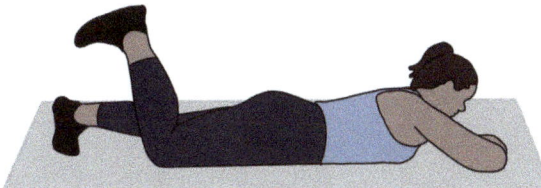

Shoulder Blade Squeezes
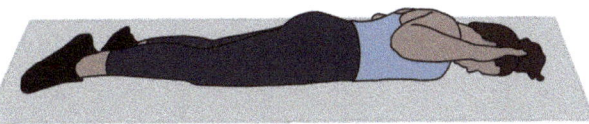

Once you are familiar with the exercises, use this as a quick reference to decrease having to flip pages as you workout.

LYING DOWN | STRETCH

Hold each stretch for 30 seconds, repeat 3 times on each side.

Hip Extension

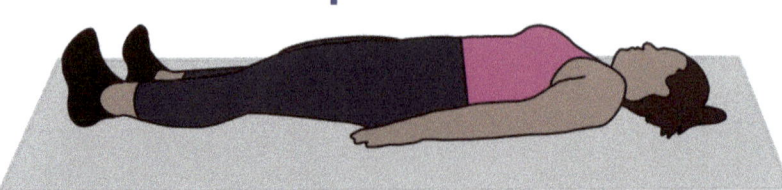
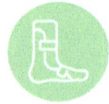

Laying on your back, straighten both legs. If able, lay one leg off the edge of the bed letting it drop towards the floor. To increase the stretch, bend your knee.
Tip: If stretching your affected side - just laying flat may feel tight. Ease into it and listen to your body. Work to slowly get further over multiple days.

Hamstring

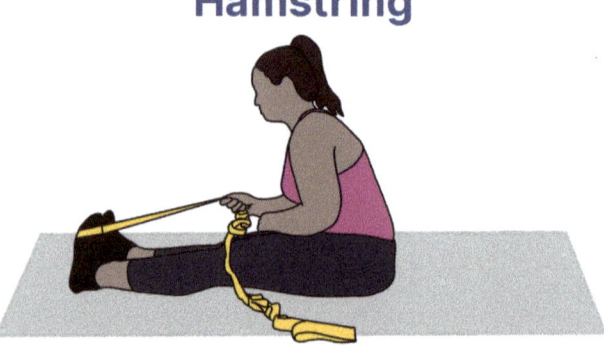
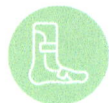

With one or both legs out in front of you, hinge forwards from the hips bringing your chest towards your toes. Try to keep your back straight.
Tip: You can use a stretching strap to help pull you forward.

Ankle Dorsiflexion

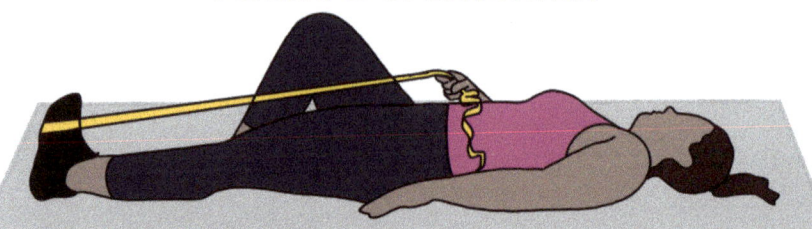

Using a stretching strap, loop one end across the ball of the foot. Pull towards you until you feel a stretch in the calf.
Tip: keeping the knee straight will help increase the stretch.
*this can be combined with the hamstring stretch to save time.

STRETCH

LYING DOWN

Hold each stretch for 30 seconds, repeat 3 times on each side.

Piriformis

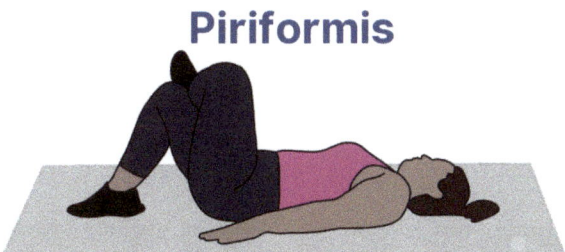
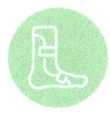

Laying on your back, bend both knees and bring one ankle across to the opposite knee. Gently press the top knee away from you, or to increase the stretch, pull the lower leg closer to you.

Tip: Keep holding the ankle to prevent the leg from falling down.

Arm Extension

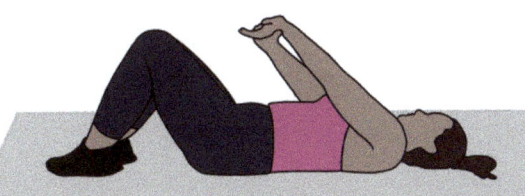
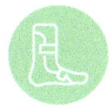

Using your opposite hand, grab your palm and extend the elbow and wrist as far straight as tolerated; The further you lower it, the more intense it will feel.

Tip: Don't grab the fingers of the side being stretched - that creates undue stress on the finger joints. Ensure you are holding and applying pressure on the palm.

Hand Opening

*Only needed if your hand tends to rest in a fisted position or feels tight.

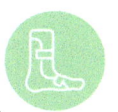
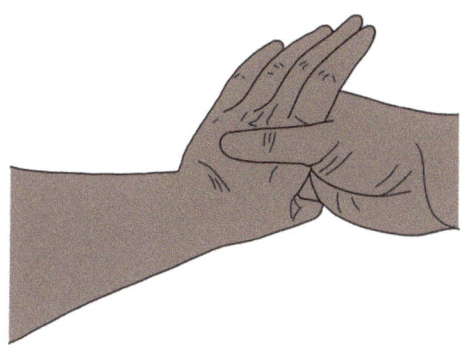

Using your unaffected side, slide 1-2 fingers along the affected palm. Gently slide out to open the fingers until you are able to get a flat palm under all your fingers and hold. Do not overstretch at the knuckles.

Tip: After stretching, attempt 10 fist openings to a splayed hand - even if just a few fingers move it's still beneficial.

> **BE COMMITTED TO YOURSELF. YOU DESERVE IT!**

SEATED
SEATED
SEATED

SEATED STRENGTH

Leg Kicks

Hamstring Curls

Hip Abductions

Core Lean Backs

Partial Stands

Shoulder Blade Squeezes

Biceps Curls

Shoulder Abductions

STRENGTH

SEATED

Leg Kicks

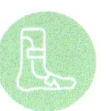

Start seated on the edge of a chair with a resistance band at your ankles. Kick one leg out extending the knee all the way straight. Hold 3 seconds. Slowly lower back.

Repeat 8-12 reps x 2 sets

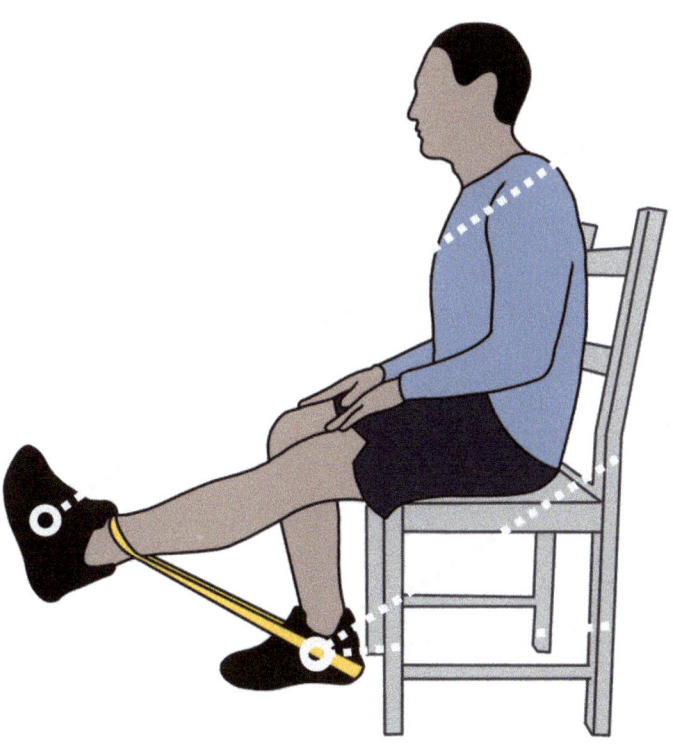

Pull the toes towards you to make the leg work harder.

Anchor the band with your heel or tie it to the chair leg.

Return the foot all the way under you each repetition.

Too Hard?
Complete the move with no resistance and as much range as you are able.

Too Easy?
Add small circles at the top range while holding.

SEATED STRENGTH

Hamstring Curls

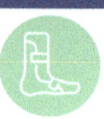

Start with a resistance band anchored in front of you. With the leg kicked out straight, the resistance band should not have slack. Bend the knee to pull the foot back underneath you. Slowly return to the starting position.

Repeat 8-12 reps x 2 sets

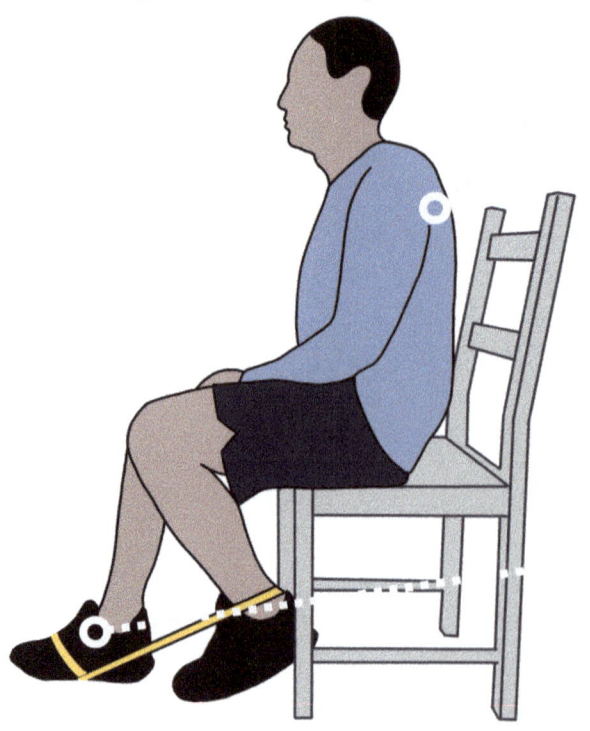

Sit up tall away from the back of the chair.

There are options for how to anchor your resistance.

Use your opposite foot, have someone hold it or tie it to a table leg.

Too Hard?
Place your foot on a pillowcase or paper plate and bend the knee to pull the foot underneath you.

Too Easy?
Add up to a 10 second hold at end range.

STRENGTH

SEATED

Hip Abductions

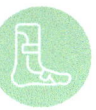

Start seated on the edge of a chair with a resistance band just above the knees. Press out with both legs as far as you can. Hold 5 seconds. Slowly return to the starting position.

Repeat 8-12 reps x 2 sets

Make sure you have good posture - sitting upright.

The closer to the edge of the chair the more range you will have.

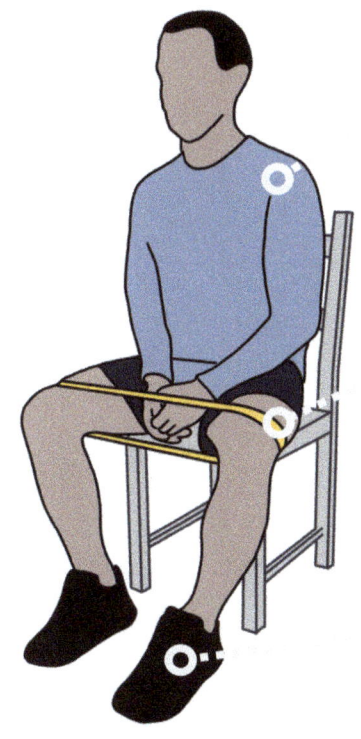

Feet should start about 6 inches apart.

Too Hard?

Perform one side at a time to focus on the movement or remove the band.

Too Easy?

Do single legs and add a lift before you move the leg outwards. Alternate sides.

SEATED STRENGTH

Core Lean Backs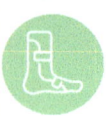

Start sitting upright on the edge of a chair. Slowly tilt back, hinging from the hips. You will feel your abdominals kicking in. Pause and return to the starting position.

Repeat 8-12 reps x 2 sets

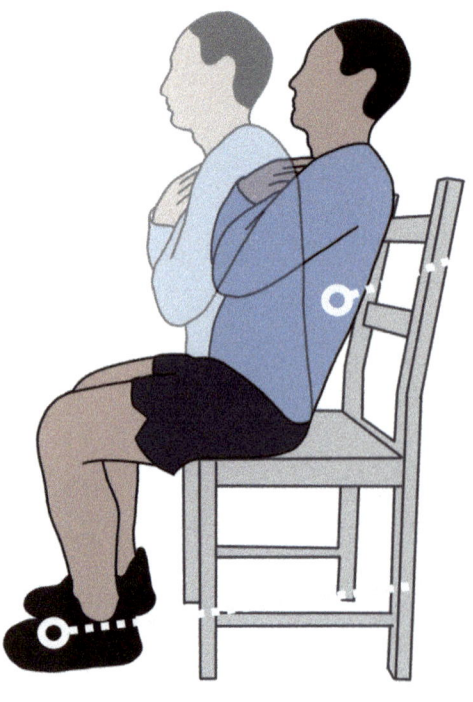

Keep breathing - do not hold your breath.

Keep a straight line at your back, don't slump.

If your feet lift off the ground, you are going too far.

Too Hard?
Start with a much smaller range, tilt back just enough to feel the abdominals kick in.

Too Easy?
Hold a hand weight against your chest and hold 5 seconds at end range.

STRENGTH

SEATED

Partial Stands

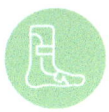

Start seated at the front edge of a sturdy chair. Make sure feet are flat on the floor. If able, place both hands on arm rests or edges of the chair as shown. Begin to press up to a partial stand using legs and arms to help. Hold up to 5 seconds then lower slowly back down.

Repeat 8-12 reps x 2 sets

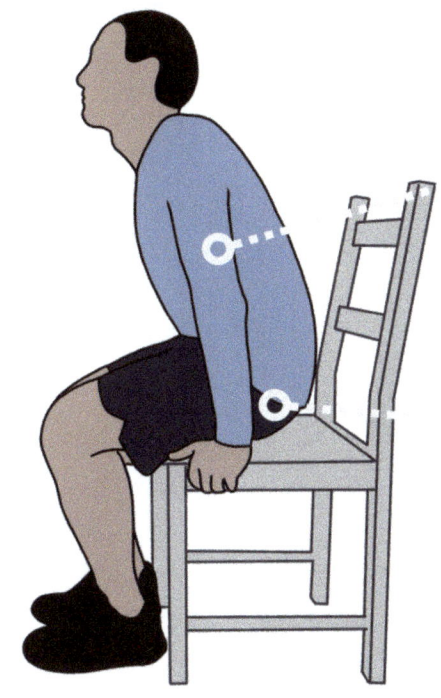

If you are in a wheelchair make sure it's locked!

If you can only position one arm to push that's ok.

You are just lifting the hips, not standing all the way.

Too Hard?
Start with glute sets - squeezing buttocks together to activate.

Too Easy?
Complete full sit to stands focusing on control.

SEATED STRENGTH

Shoulder Blade Squeezes

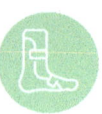

Start seated upright on the edge of a sturdy chair. Hold a resistance band across both hands, with palms facing up. Squeeze the shoulder blades back and together while separating your hands.

Repeat 8-12 reps x 2 sets

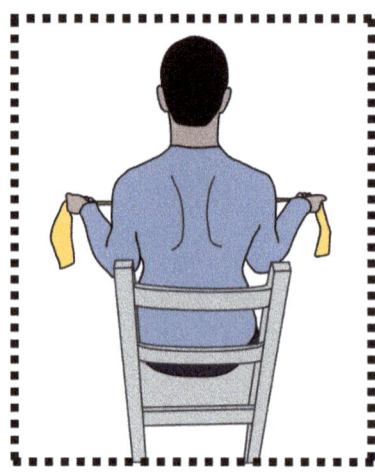
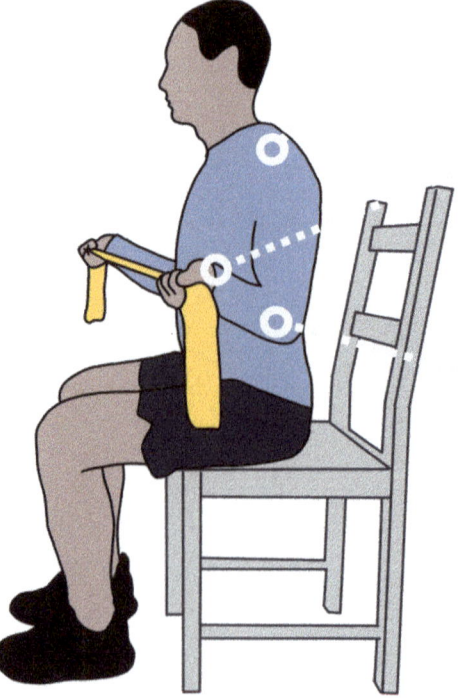

Starting posture is key - keep your head up and shoulders down.

Thumbs should be pointing outwards the entire time.

Keep your elbows close to the body.

Too Hard?
Perform with no resistance focusing on the squeeze between the shoulder blades.

Too Easy?
Start with your hands closer for more resistance and hold at end range.

STRENGTH

SEATED

Biceps Curls

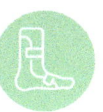

Start sitting at the edge of a chair holding a hand weight in each hand. Arms start extended down at your sides. Bend at the elbow lifting the weights towards your shoulders then slowly lower back down.

Repeat 8-12 reps x 2 sets

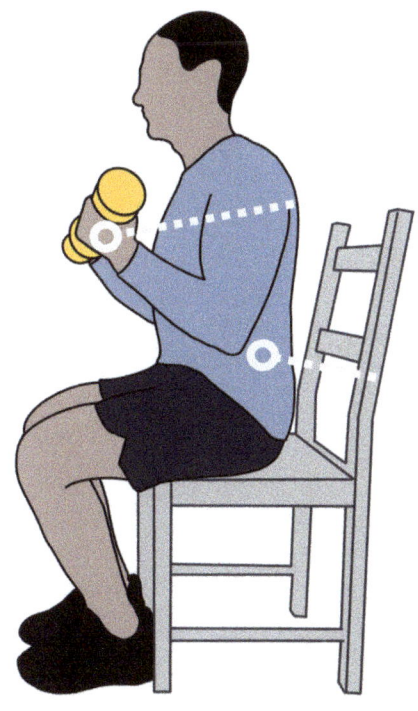

Skip this move if your elbow is stuck in a bent position. Focus on straightening.

Keep palms facing the ceiling as you bend the elbows

Ensure good posture throughout - no leaning back.

Too Hard?
Perform one arm at a time and/or with no weights.

Too Easy?
Add a punch forwards at end range with each rep.

56

SEATED STRENGTH

Shoulder Abductions

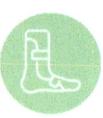

Start seated with a hand weight in each hand. Keeping the elbows straight (as much as possible), lift hands up to shoulder height. Slowly lower back down.

Repeat 8-12 reps x 2 sets

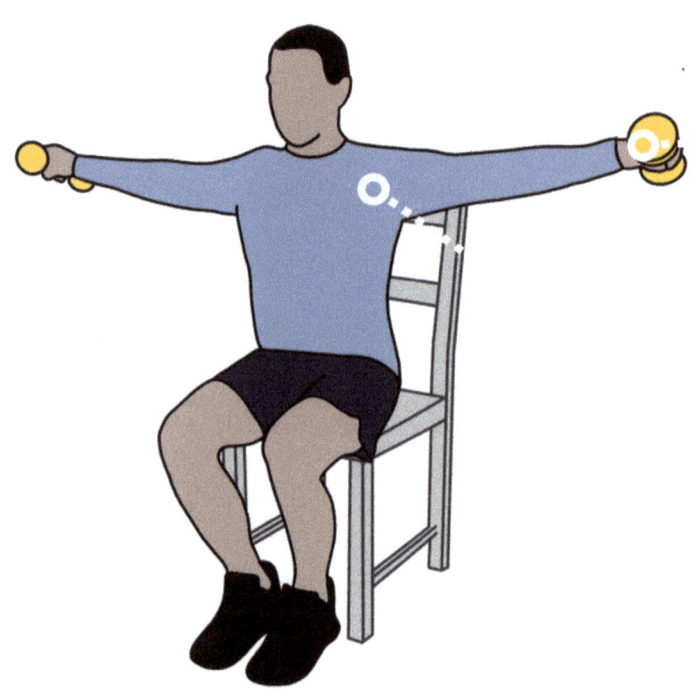

- Ensure good posture throughout.
- Palms should be facing the ground as you lift up.
- Don't let your shoulders shrug up towards your ears.

Too Hard?
Perform with no resistance and if needed bend the elbow before lifting the arm out.

Too Easy?
Increase resistance and add a 5 second hold.

Seated

Quick View

Leg Kicks | Hamstring Curls | Hip Abductions | Core Lean Backs

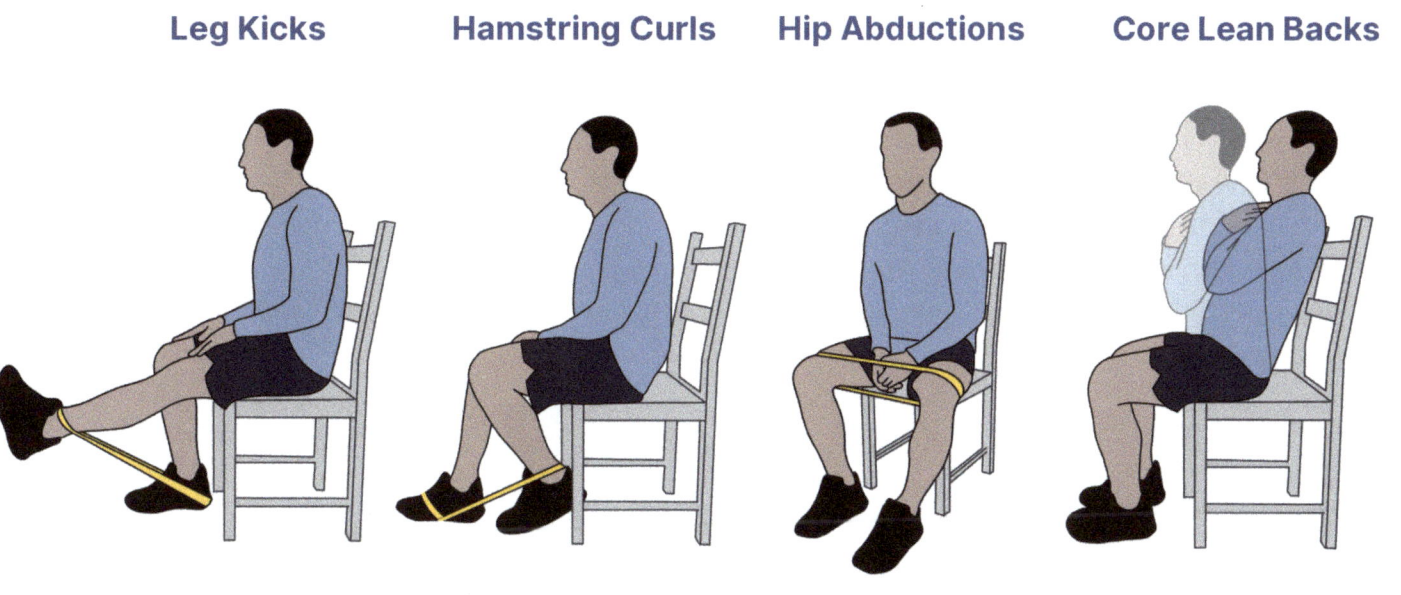

Partial Stands | Shoulder Blade Squeezes | Biceps Curls | Shoulder Abductions

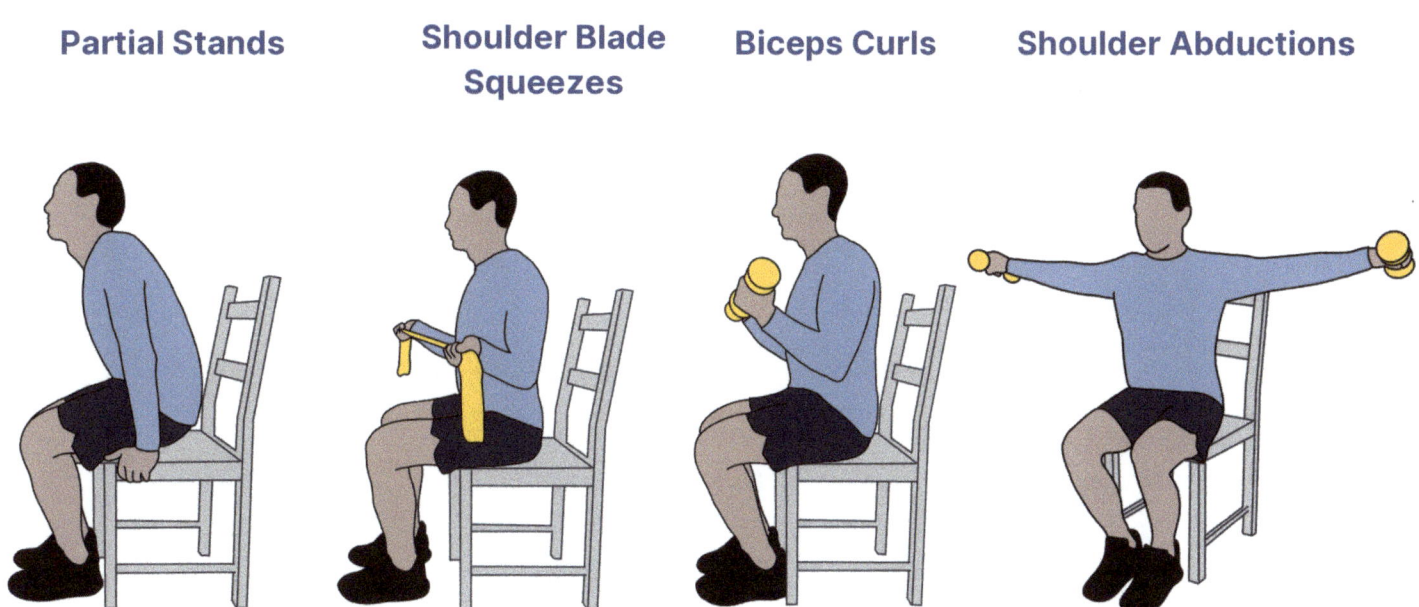

Once you are familiar with the exercises, use this as a quick reference to decrease having to flip pages as you workout.

SEATED STRETCH

Hold each stretch for 30 seconds, repeat 3 times on each side.

Hamstring and Calf

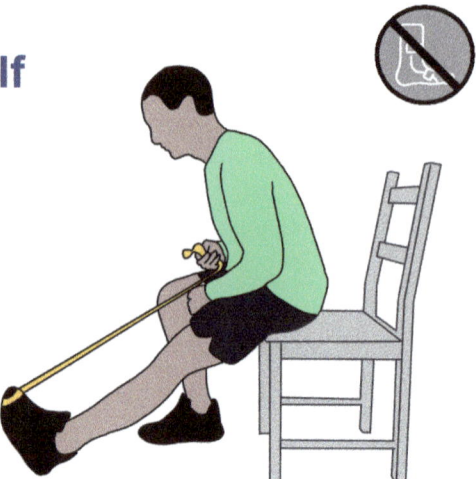

Sit with one leg extended out and toes pulled back toward you. Fold forward, feeling a pull up the back of your straight leg.
Tip: You can use a stretching strap to help pull you forward. The strap is NOT to lean back against. Make sure the heel stays on the ground.

Piriformis Figure-Four

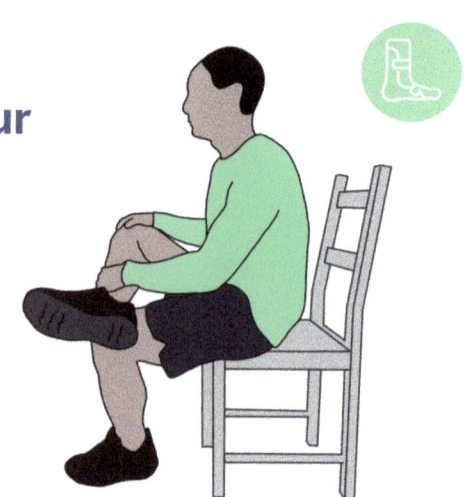

Sit in a figure-four position with one ankle on the opposite knee. Fold forward as you feel a stretch through the hips.
Tip: Keep your hand on the ankle to prevent it from sliding off.

Elbow and Wrist Extension Combo

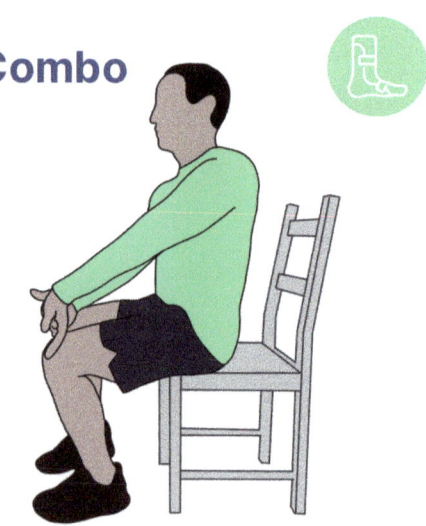

Holding the palm of one hand with the opposite hand's fingers, extend the wrist as you extend the elbow straight.
Tip: Go as far as tolerated and hold. If needed, focus on just elbow extension first then add in the wrist extension once improved.

STRETCH

SEATED

Hold each stretch for 30 seconds, repeat 3 times on each side.

Hip Flexor

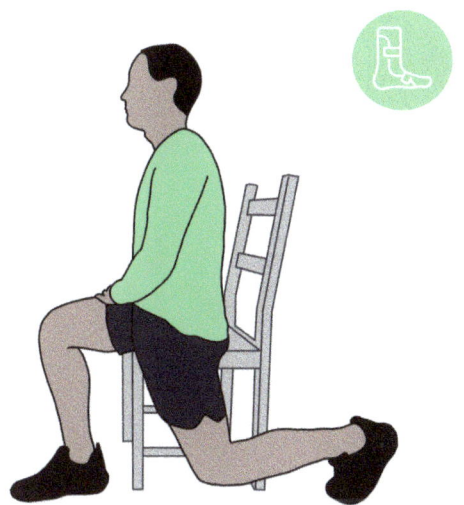

Sit to the side of a chair and pull one leg back alongside the chair pointing the knee downwards. Lift your chest up and lean back to increase the stretch.

Tip: If you don't have an armless chair, tuck your foot under your chair from the front, dropping your knee towards the floor. You will have to lean back a bit more to feel as much of a stretch. Always keep a grip on the chair to not slide off!

Trunk Extensions

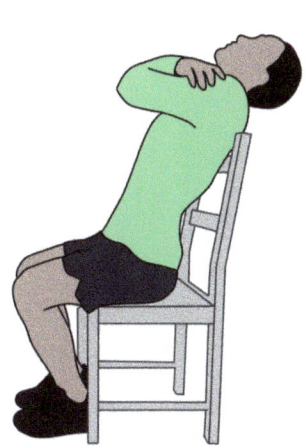

Hug yourself at the shoulders feeling a stretch between the shoulder blades. If tolerated, extend back lifting the elbows to the ceiling and head looking up.

Tip: Make sure you are seated back in the chair against a backrest that is ideally just below shoulder height for optimal stretch.

Hand Opening

*Only needed if your hand tends to rest in a fisted position or feels tight.

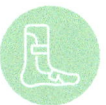

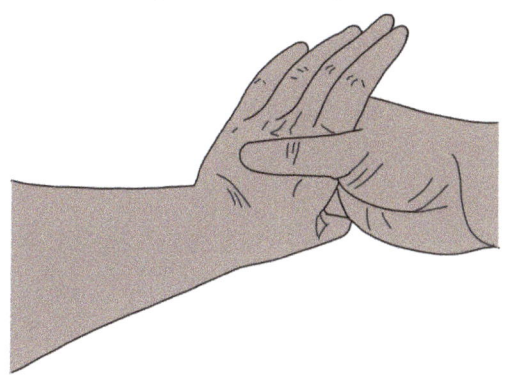

Using your unaffected side, slide 1-2 fingers along the affected palm. Gently slide out to open the fingers until you are able to get a flat palm under all your fingers and hold. Do not overstretch at the knuckles.

Tip: After stretching, attempt 10 fist openings to a splayed hand - even if just a few fingers move it's still beneficial.

YOU ARE AMAZING. NOW PROVE IT TO YOURSELF.

STANDING

STANDING STRENGTH

Heel Rises

Toe Rises

Squats

Banded Hip Circles

Hamstring Curls

Biceps Curl and Punch

Bent Over Rows

Triceps Kickbacks

STRENGTH

STANDING

Heel Rises

Stand with feet flat. Slowly raise your heels off the ground lifting yourself straight up. Lower back down controlled.

Repeat 15-20 reps x 2 sets
*note the higher reps on this move

Look straight ahead, not at your feet.

Do not bend your knees.

Keep pressure into your big toes to prevent the ankles from rolling out.

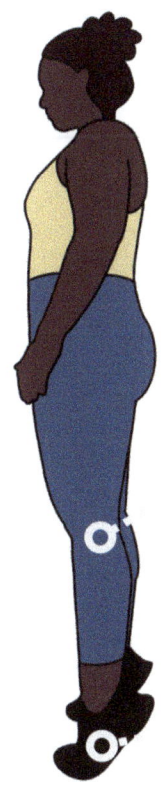

Too Hard?
Perform one side at a time, keeping the opposite foot on the ground.

Too Easy?
Perform in single leg stance.

64

STANDING STRENGTH

Toe Rises

Stand with feet flat. Slowly raise the toes and balls of your feet off the ground. Lower back down controlled.

Repeat 15-20 reps x 2 sets
*note the higher reps on this move

Look straight ahead, not at your feet.

Do not let your hips tilt back. All motion is at the ankle.

Be near something sturdy to grab for balance!

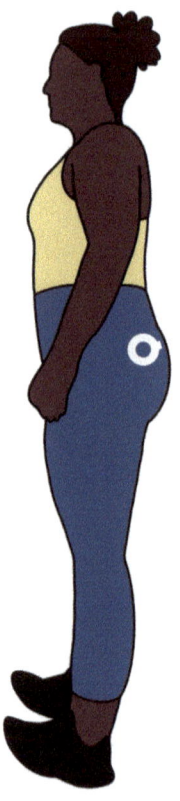

Too Hard?
Perform one side at a time, keeping the opposite foot on the ground.

Too Easy?
Perform in single leg stance.

STRENGTH

STANDING

Squats

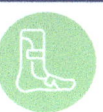

Start standing tall with feet hip width apart. Slowly lower your hips as if to sit in a chair behind you. Pause at the lowest point you can hold then return to full standing.

Repeat 8-12 reps x 2 sets

Keep your chest facing forward, not to the floor. If you cannot, you are going too far.

Hips need to go back, not your knees forward.

Have a chair behind you in case you go down too far.

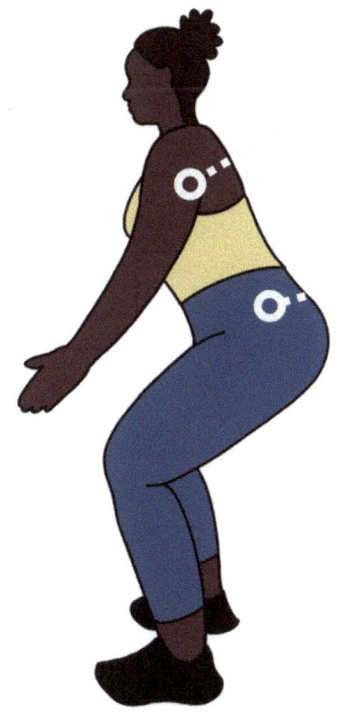

Too Hard?
Hold onto a sturdy support while performing a smaller squat movement.

Too Easy?
Perform in a single leg stance with one leg out in front of you.

STANDING

STRENGTH

Banded Hip Circles

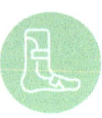

Start with a resistance band around your legs, just above the knees. Stand in a slight crouch so both knees have a soft bend. Draw a circle with one leg by pressing forward, to the side, and behind. Return to starting position.

Repeat 8-12 reps x 2 sets

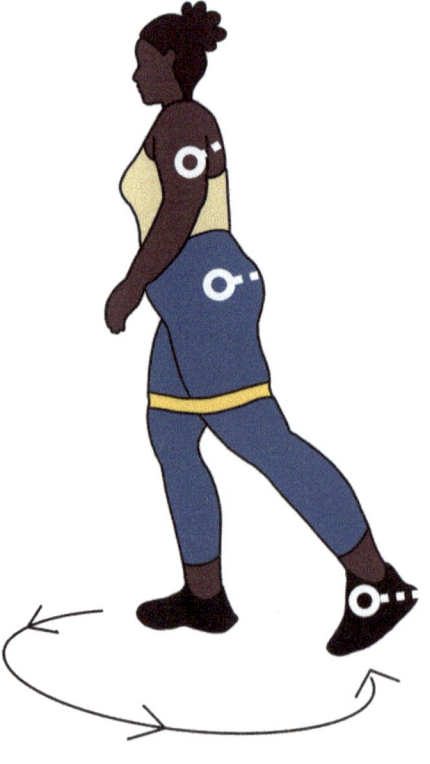

Keep your chest forward and upper body still. All motion is at the hip.

It's normal for your standing hip to get tired. It's holding your whole body up!

Flex up at the ankle - don't point the foot during the movement.

Too Hard?
Complete the movement without resistance bands.

Too Easy?
Lower the resistance band to the ankles.

67

STRENGTH

STANDING

Hamstring Curls

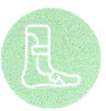

Start with a resistance band around the ankles (or use an ankle weight). Bend one knee, bringing the foot back towards the buttocks until you reach a 90 degree angle ("L" shaped). Slowly lower to the starting position.

Repeat 8-12 reps x 2 sets

Keep your trunk up tall throughout the exercise.

Do not let your knee move forward - the thighs should stay together.

Tuck the band under your heel to prevent it from sliding up as you move.

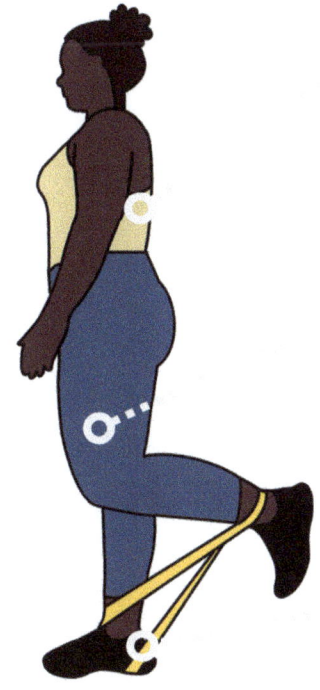

Too Hard?
Perform with no resistance, focusing on range and posture.

Too Easy?
Add a hold at end range or increase resistance.

STANDING STRENGTH

Biceps Curl and Punch

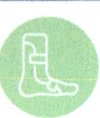

Start holding hand weights down at your sides with elbows straight. Bend the elbows, bringing your hands towards your shoulders. Once there, press out to a forward punch. Return the hands to shoulders then slowly lower to the starting position.

Repeat 8-12 reps x 2 sets

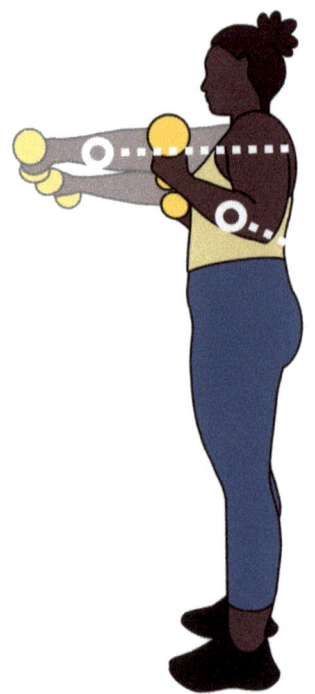

Keep the trunk still, make the arms do the work.

Palms face your body during the curl then toward the floor as you punch.

Elbows stay close to the body during the curl portion.

Too Hard?
Perform with no resistance and/or one arm at a time.

Too Easy?
Add a hold at the punch and flip the palms up and back down before completing the movement.

STRENGTH

STANDING

Bent Over Rows

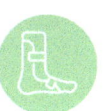

Start holding hand weights while in a forward leaning position. Arms start out towards the ground with palms facing each other. Lift your elbows up toward the ceiling while squeezing your shoulder blades together. Lower your arms back down slowly.

Repeat 8-12 reps x 2 sets

Keep your head and neck in neutral, looking at the floor out in front of you.

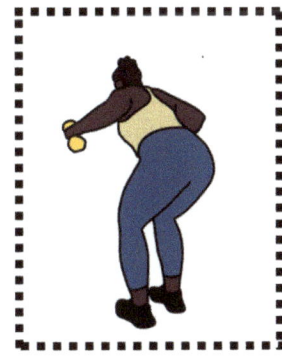

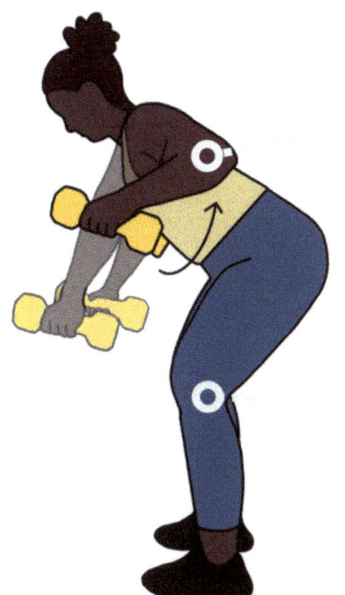

Elbows will move away from the body.

Keep a soft bend in both knees to take pressure off the low back.

Too Hard?
Perform the move with no resistance, focusing on technique.

Too Easy?
Increase the resistance and hold at end range 5 seconds.

70

STANDING STRENGTH

Triceps Kickbacks

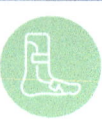

Start holding hand weights while in a forward leaning position. Arms start tucked close to the body and elbows bent to 90 degrees. Slowly extend the arms back, straightening the elbows while bringing the hands towards the ceiling behind you.

Repeat 8-12 reps x 2 sets

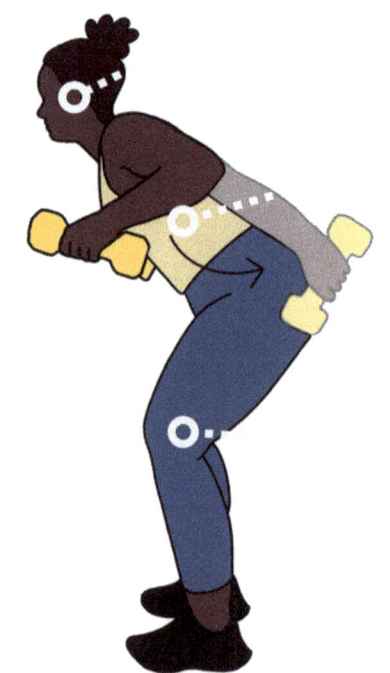

Keep your head and neck in neutral, looking at the floor out in front of you.

The further you lean forwards to start, the harder it is.

Keep a soft bend in both knees to take pressure off the low back.

Too Hard?
Perform with no resistance and/or one arm at a time.

Too Easy?
Add a 3 count pulse at the end range - lifting the extended arm just a little further to the ceiling.

Standing
Quick View

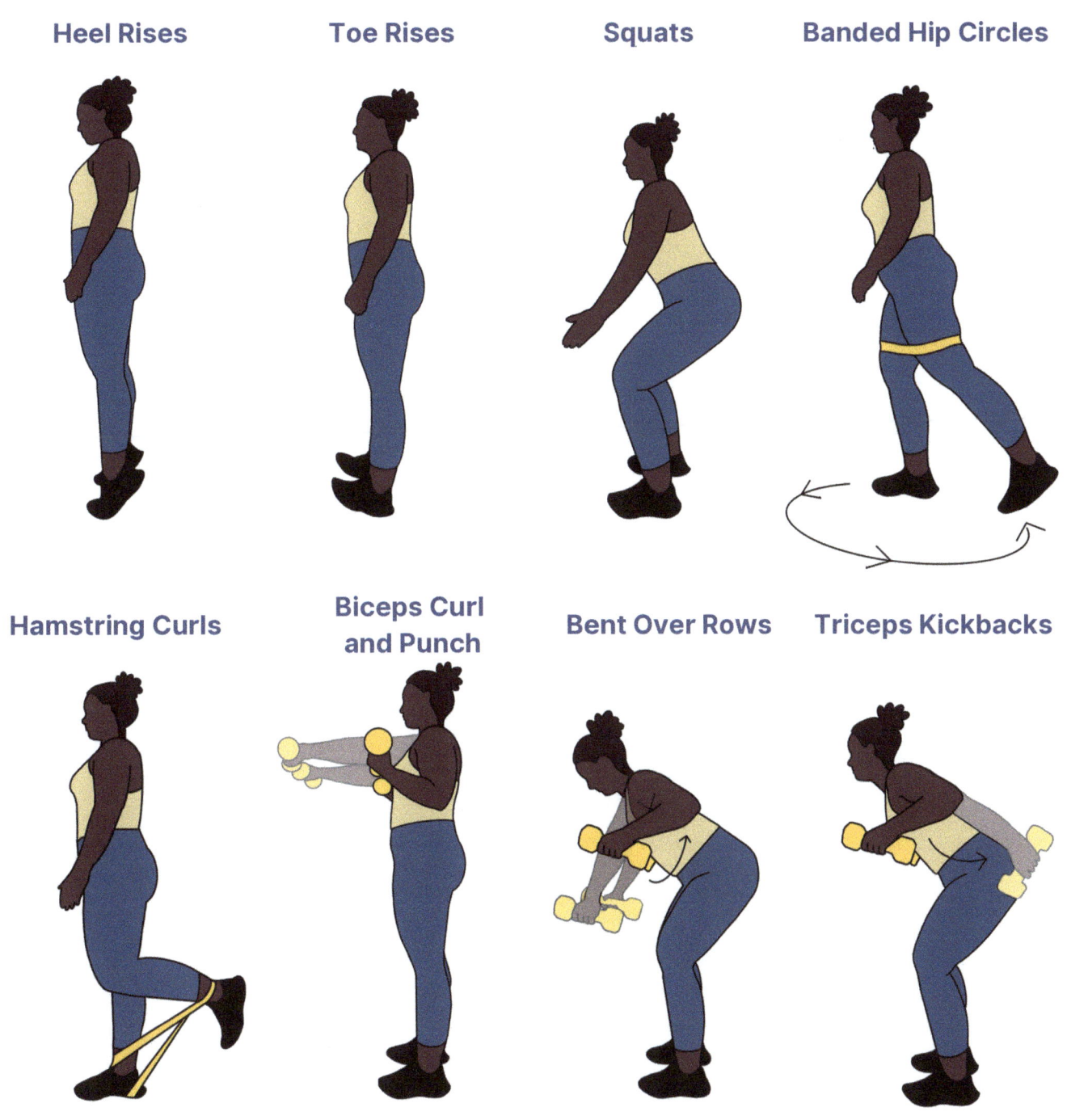

Once you are familiar with the exercises, use this as a quick reference to decrease having to flip pages as you workout.

STANDING STRETCH

Hold each stretch for 30 seconds, repeat 3 times on each side.

Hold on during all standing stretching. The goal is to have the stretching leg relaxed which you cannot do if it is balancing you.

Many stretches include using the bottom 2-3 stairs. If you do not have access to a step or stairs, you can use a sturdy ottoman, step stool, etc. Just make sure you have something sturdy to hold.

Calf

Facing a wall, set the front of your foot on the vertical surface with your heel on the floor. Keeping your knee straight, lean your body forwards creating a stretch up the back of your lower leg. You can repeat with the knee bent for a variation to hit deeper muscles.

Tip: You can also use a wedge, small block or wall to brace against.

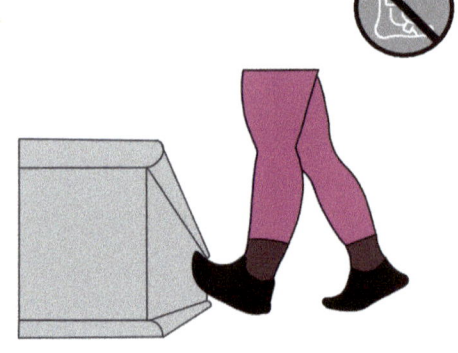

Hamstrings

With one leg on a step in front of you, hinge forwards from the hips bringing your shoulders towards your toes.

Tip: Keep your shoulders squared. Without a step, you can place one leg forward on the floor but you will need to hinge further.

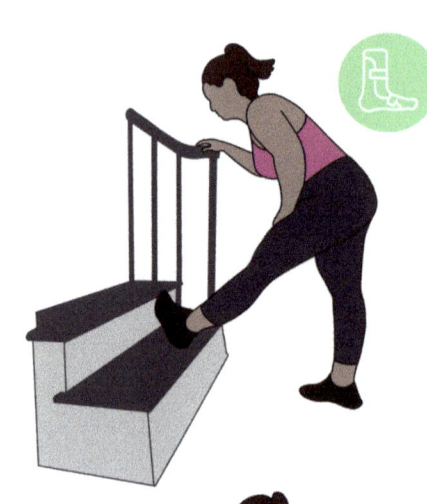

Hip Complex

Placing your foot flat on a 2nd or 3rd step, lunge forwards keeping your back knee straight and chest upright.

Tip: The further you lunge forward and lean the trunk back at the same time the more stretch you will feel.

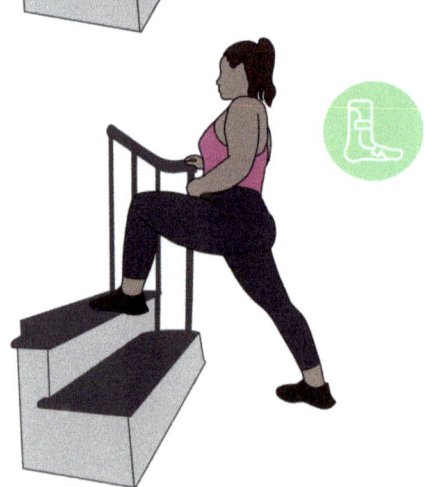

STRETCH

STANDING

Hold each stretch for 30 seconds, repeat 3 times on each side.

Standing Elbow and Wrist Extension Combo

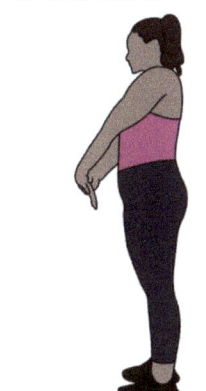
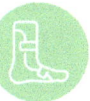

Holding the palm of one hand with the opposite hand's fingers, extend the wrist as you extend the elbow.

Tip: Go as far as tolerated and hold. If needed, focus on just elbow extension first then add in the wrist extension once improved.

Doorway Pec Stretch

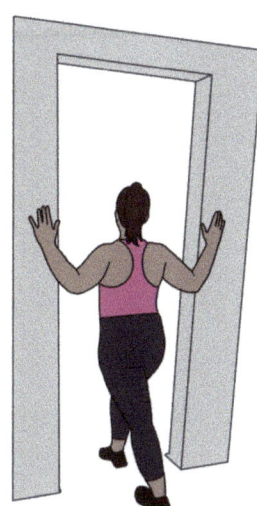
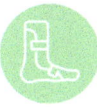

Facing an open doorway, place your palms on either side of the door frame at chest height. Step through the doorway with one foot and lean your chest forwards feeling the pull across your chest.

Tip: Variation in your hand height will change the pull - find the height that feels like a good stretch to you. Lower towards the waist is usually less intense. Higher to head level is more intense.
*Never press through sharp shooting pains in the shoulder. If there is pain, stop to reposition. If pain persists, stop and seek a medical professional.

Hand Opening

*Only needed if your hand tends to rest in a fisted position or feels tight.

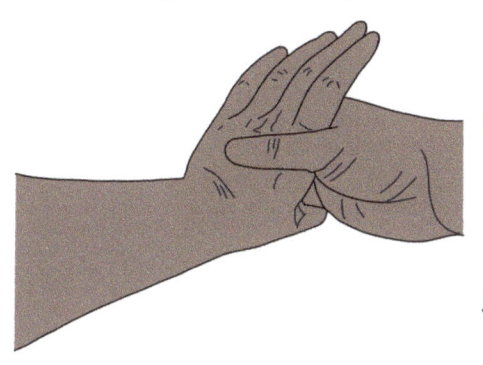

Using your unaffected side, slide 1-2 fingers along the affected palm. Gently slide out to open the fingers until you are able to get a flat palm under all your fingers and hold. Do not overstretch at the knuckles.

Tip: After stretching, attempt 10 fist openings to a splayed hand - even if just a few fingers move it's still beneficial.

74

A note about

BALANCE

Balance will improve if you use minimal hand contact as you get stronger. HOLD ON for initial trials. Some days you may have more or less energy, adjust your challenges appropriately.

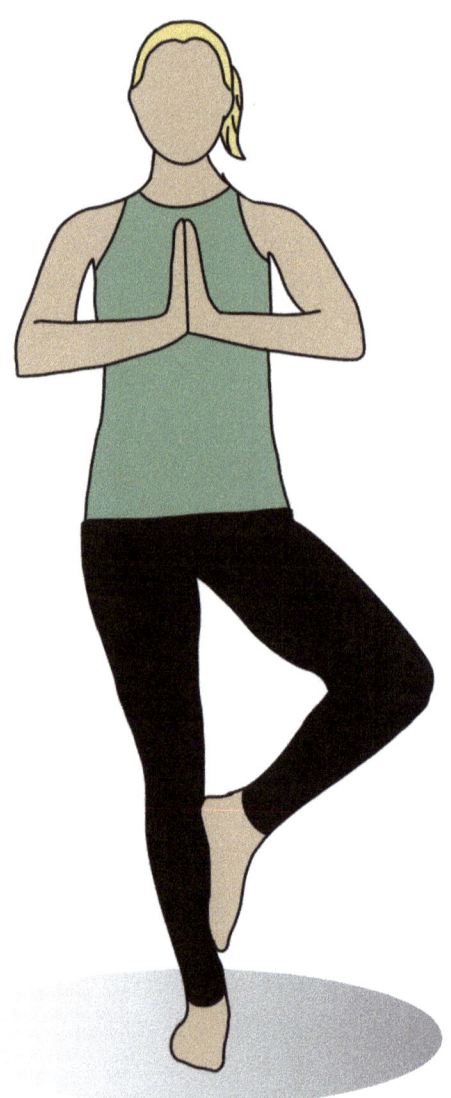

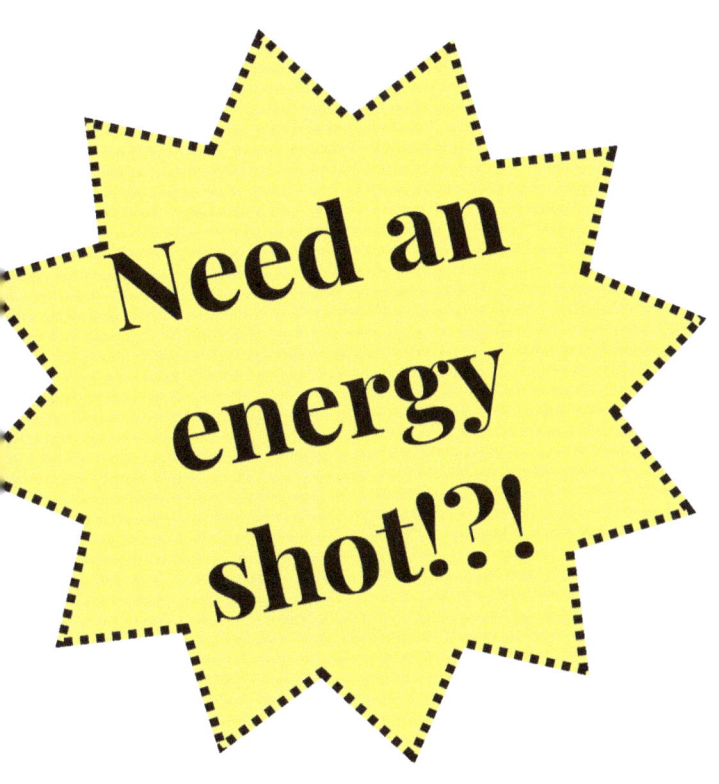

Energy Shot! Feeling tired or sluggish? Don't do nothing! Do this 5 minute energy boosting routine.

Pick your position, then **perform 3 rounds of 20 seconds for each move.** Rest up to 1 minute between moves.

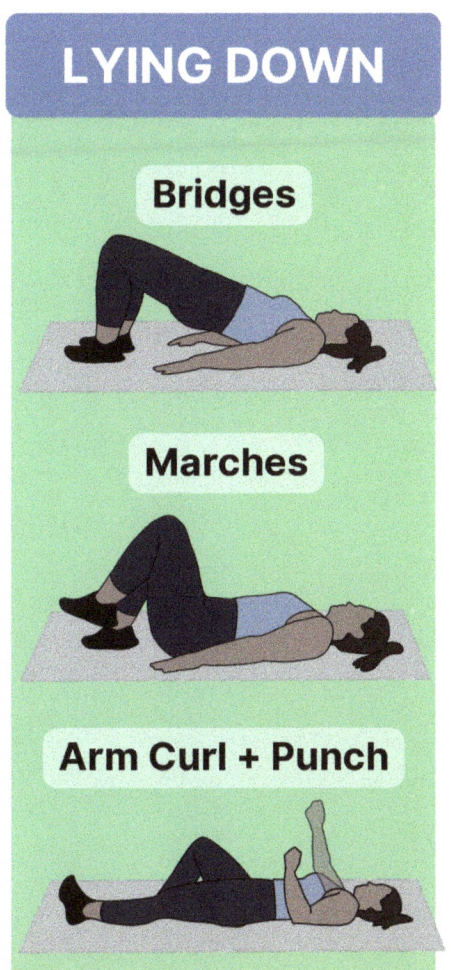
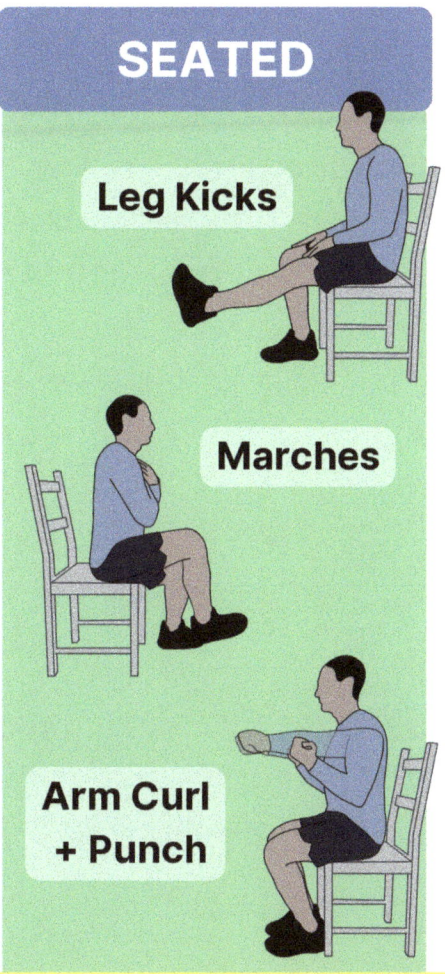
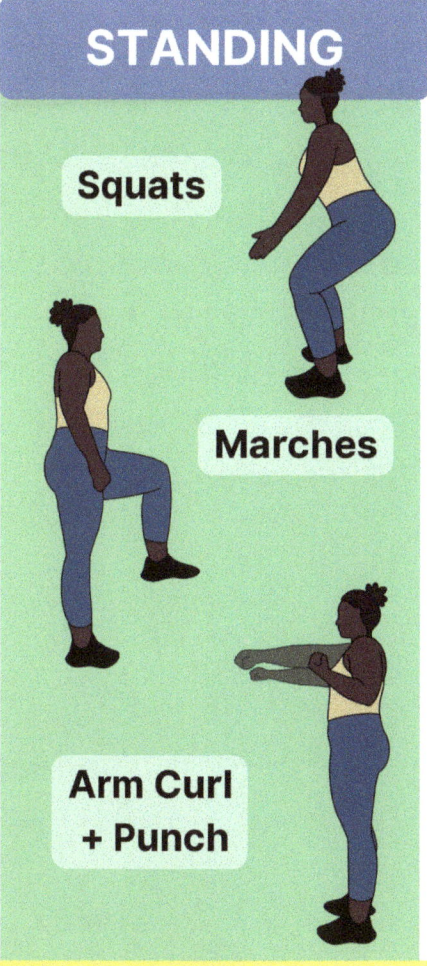

Feeling revived? Keep going and head to your complete workout.
Still tired? That's OK, at least you got the blood flowing. Try again later.

REST DAYS

Usually my job consists of trying to encourage people to move and exercise. There are some days when it is important to know when exercise is *not* the best answer.

In general, you do want one to two rest days per week. A rest day does not mean you don't leave your bed or couch. It means no strenuous activities or purposefully fatiguing exercise. You should still be moving around for your daily tasks as much as able. Light walks are great on rest days. Consider it to be "active rest". Your joints still need to move every day or you will feel worse.

ILLNESS

When you are sick, that is not the time to push the resistance training. Fighting an illness takes a lot of internal energy and you want your body to prioritize your immune system the best it can. Depending on the severity of your cold, flu, etc. active rest may still be appropriate as long as it feels safe. If not, it's okay to take a day or two to recover. Make sure you are helping your body to fight back in other ways such as increasing hydration, extra fruits and vegetables that are full of immune boosting nutrients, and proper sleep.

LISTEN TO YOUR BODY

You know your body the best. Always seek immediate medical attention if you ever feel something is wrong or if you have signs of a new stroke. Use the acronym **BE FAST** from the American Stroke Association:

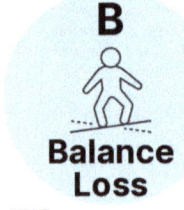
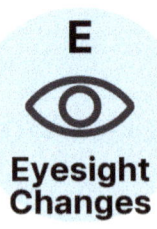
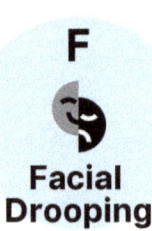
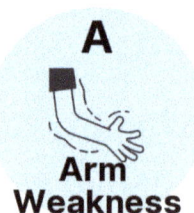
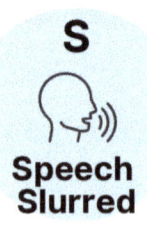

MAKE IT ALL MATTER!

The point of all of these exercises and wellness tips is not about how they will make you look. Getting and feeling stronger builds confidence and drastically improves outlook on life. It's all about improving how you feel moving around with daily activities and hobbies. Finding ways to use your new found strength will help daily movements feel easier and increase overall activity levels. Below are some ways to incorporate your strength and ways to work in extra exercises throughout your day.

Lying down in bed? Tighten your core muscles before movements like rolling over or bridging hips to dress.

Seated? Tighten your core muscles while sitting up with your best possible posture (away from the chair back) during daily tasks such as eating a meal, reaching out to grab an object or set something down.
If you aren't using it - where is that affected arm hanging out? Make sure it has proper support.

Standing in line? That's your cue to check your posture! Head up, shoulder blades pulled back, core engaged and a soft bend in your knees.
What about throwing in a few heel raises while you hold that shopping cart? I promise no one will notice.

Waiting on the microwave? Perfect! You have 30-60 seconds to do some toe rises or leg kicks.

You've been working on those squats or partial stands, so getting up is getting easier. Great! Use that renewed skill to get up for a drink of water rather than asking a family member to bring you one. This works best when you communicate your goals and motivations to your family. Work with them to find safe options where you can do more and so they know when you would and *would not* like help.

CAREGIVER NOTES

If you are at a level of still needing assistance to move parts of your body you can still participate with much of this guide, you may just need assist from family, friends or a caregiver. The notes below are to help them better help you.

Better quality of movements leads to better results. Take your time to do it right.

Listen to the person you are helping. Ask for cues on too far, not enough, help less, etc. Pay attention to facial cues like grimacing, especially if speech is affected.

Be mindful of decreased sensation which can be present after stroke. They may not feel the discomfort but being too aggressive can still trigger spasm or cause injury.

Support the limbs closer to the trunk for more control. Example: if helping to stretch an arm over head - support closer to the armpit with a second hand near the wrist.

Never hyperextend joints, this can lead to further injury.

Help stabilize non-moving parts such as keeping legs from falling to the side or sliding out in bridges.

> **Move slowly through stretches. Speed can trigger reflexive spasms which are counterproductive.**

> **When you are assisting with strength moves, do the bare minimum. You are only there to make up for what they can't do; not to make it easy.**

> **Watch your own body mechanics. You can't help others if you don't help yourself. Make sure to sit at optimal heights rather than bending over, or sit closer so you don't have to reach as far.**

> **Watch your hands! Pokey fingers hurt. Make sure you use a broad grip any time you are holding onto them.**

> **Use this as time to connect. Chatting and making the time fun improves the likelihood of making it a habit.**

> **Remember, hands are healing. Just having the extra mindful touch can do wonders for feeling better.**

> **Join in! You don't have to be hands-on to help. Exercise is always more fun with a buddy!**

Remember, a supportive family or caregiver is a blessing. Accepting a little (or a lot) of help can be difficult. Often people are too proud to ask for help, feel like a burden, or feel that the help they get "isn't the same" as a professional. Make sure you share these tips so those assisting you can be safe and effective.

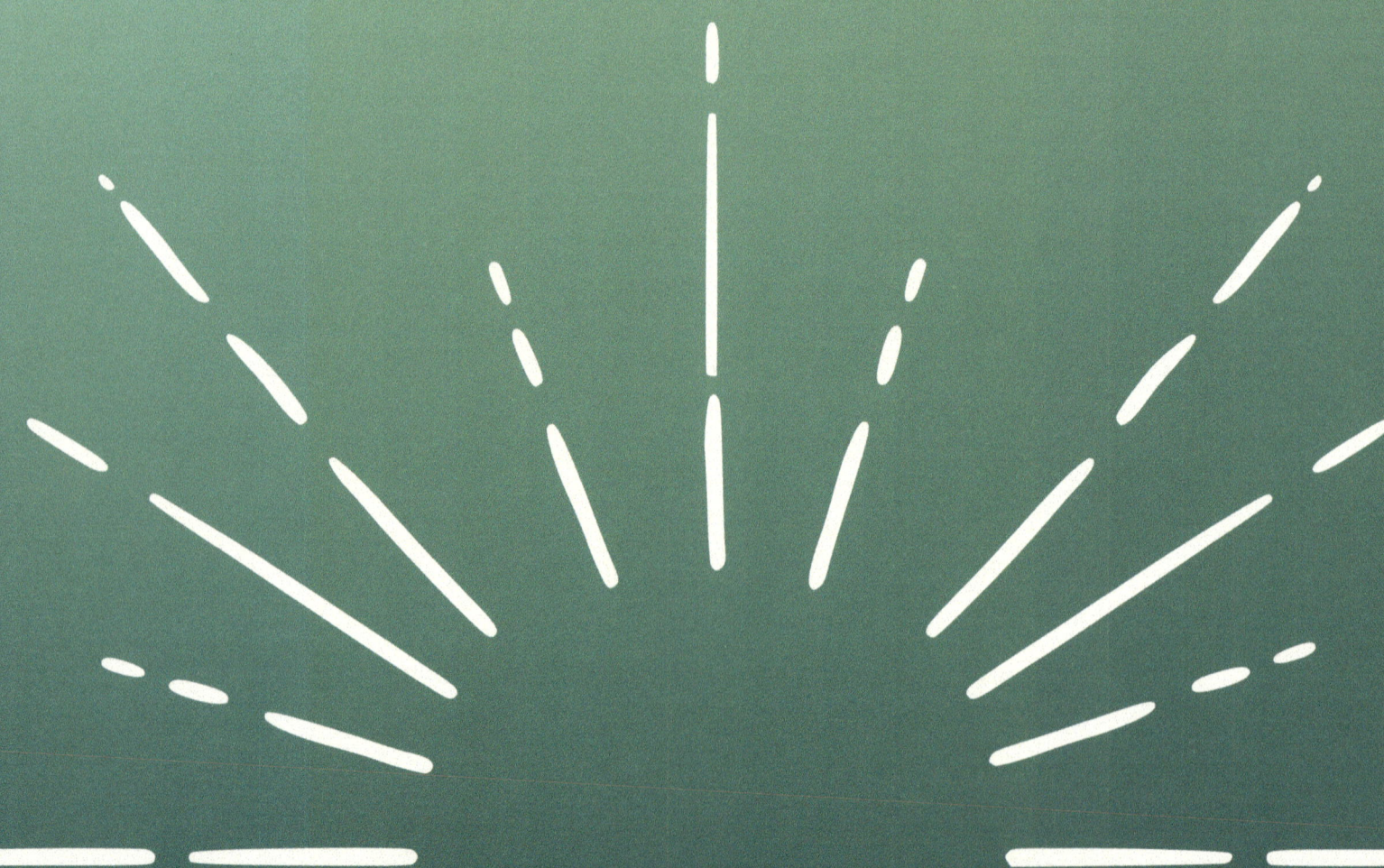

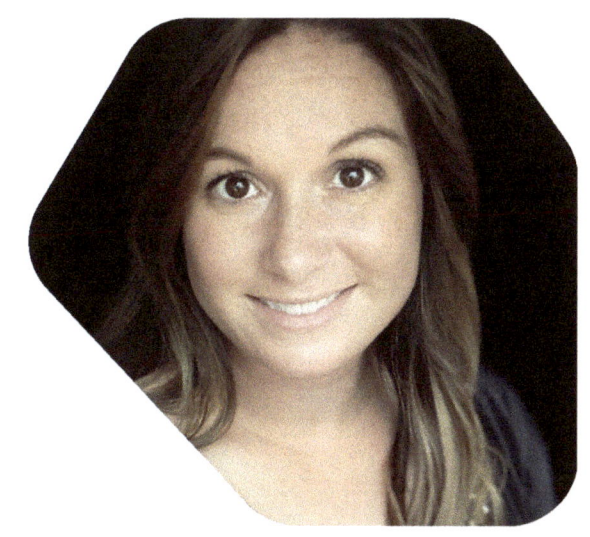

ABOUT THE AUTHOR

Dr. Sarah Stollberg, PT, DPT graduated from Marquette University with a Doctorate of Physical Therapy and Bachelors in Exercise Science. For over a decade she has worked one-on-one with patients after stroke in a variety of settings including acute care, transitional care, short and long term nursing homes and outpatient therapy.

"I have worked a wide range of settings, seeing what post-stroke care looks like from onset to many years out. I noticed I could make the biggest impact where there was a huge gap in care - after discharge! I hope this guide gives you the confidence and knowledge to keep moving long after you hit "max rehab potential".
~Dr. Sarah Stollberg, PT, DPT

Common Knowledge PT, LLC is a publishing company on a mission to make health and wellness education more...common! Check out the latest resources and supplements at the links below.

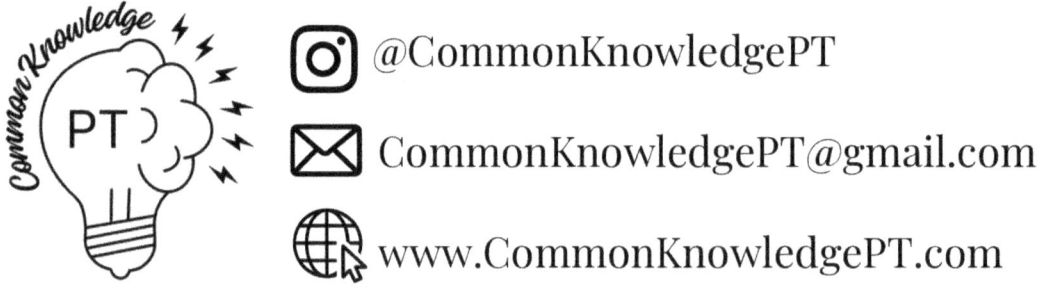

@CommonKnowledgePT

CommonKnowledgePT@gmail.com

www.CommonKnowledgePT.com

www.ingramcontent.com/pod-product-compliance
Lightning Source LLC
Chambersburg PA
CBHW042358030426
42337CB00032B/5149